DANCE THERAPY

DANCE THERAPY
Theory and Application

By

LILJAN ESPENAK, M.A., DTR
Assistant Professor
New York Medical College
Director of Postgraduate Training in Dance Therapy
Mental Retardation Institute
Valhalla, New York

and

Developmental Disabilities Clinic, Flower Hospital
New York, New York

With Forewords by

Alexandra Adler, M.D.
Medical Director, Alfred Adler Mental Hygiene Clinic
Clinical Professor of Psychiatry
New York University, School of Medicine
New York, New York

and

Alexander Lowen, M.D.
Executive Director, Institute for Bioenergetic Analysis
New York, New York

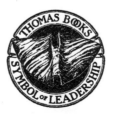

CHARLES C THOMAS · PUBLISHER
Springfield · Illinois · U.S.A.

Published and Distributed Throughout the World by
CHARLES C THOMAS • PUBLISHER
Bannerstone House
301-327 East Lawrence Avenue, Springfield, Illinois, U.S.A.

© *1981, by* CHARLES C THOMAS • PUBLISHER
ISBN 0-398-04110-5
Library of Congress Catalog Card Number: 80-16587

With THOMAS BOOKS *careful attention is given to all details of
manufacturing and design. It is the Publisher's desire to present books
that are satisfactory as to their physical qualities and artistic possibilities
and appropriate for their particular use.* THOMAS BOOKS *will be
true to those laws of quality that assure a good name and good will.*

Library of Congress Cataloging in Publication Data

Espenak, Liljan.
    Dance therapy.

    Bibliography: p.
    Includes index.
    1. Dance therapy. I. Title. [DNLM: 1. Dance
therapy. WM450.5.D2 E77d]
RC489.D3E86   616.89'1655   80-16587
ISBN 0-398-04110-5

Printed in the United States of America
W-2

to Doctor Harold Michal-Smith
my advisor and friend

FOREWORD

T WENTY YEARS AGO the author of this book entered the Adler Institute as a student and as an émigrée from Europe, where she had been both a performer and teacher of the dance. In this earlier work abroad, Mrs. Espenak had become intensely aware of the relationship between body and mind, as expressed in body behaviors and body movement, and had begun to focus in her work and in her study upon the reciprocities of this interaction. This growing awareness stimulated her interest in psychology and psychiatry and constituted the beginning of what was to become her lifework in dance therapy.

During the ensuing years of study in the approaches of the major schools of related professional disciplines, Liljan Espenak found herself drawn to certain major concepts in Adlerian psychology because a number of elements in our approach had confirmed and supplemented her own experience and theoretical understanding of psychomotor interaction. She perceived that a therapeutic approach, derived from the Adlerian concepts, could be developed and applied effectively to her own work in the treatment of body behaviors.

This rapport with the work of Alfred Adler is reflected in her own professional approach, particularly in regard to those aspects of Alderian psychology which focus on biological and physiological affect in psychological development. Adler's early book, *Study of Organ Inferiority and Its Psychical Compensation* published in 1907, foreshadowed his introduction of a new dimension in psychological thought to clinical medicine.

It is particularly interesting that this psychosomatic view—and other elements in Adler's theoretical work, such as the significance of social feeling as a factor in healthy personality development and the role of memory in life-style formations—appeared to relate closely to Mrs. Espenak's personal experience and observation as dancer and teacher. She was, at the time of her initial immersion in Adler's theories, just beginning to structure her theoretical platform for psychomotor therapy, with the conviction that a psychotherapeutic approach, derived in part from Adler's concepts, could be developed and applied effectively to the treatment of body behaviors.

Mrs. Espenak thus studied with us at the Alfred Adler Institute, New York, during which time she developed her schematic structure of psychomotor theory. Her first applications as a therapist began in 1964 at the University Affiliated Mental Retardation Clinic at Flower-Fifth Avenue Hospitals. After she completed studies at our Institute, she introduced dance therapy to our Rehabilitation Social Club, which we conduct with a view toward rehabilitation of released former mental patients who live in the community and become patients of the Alfred Adler Mental Health Clinic.

Overall, then, it is now some fifteen years that Mrs. Espenak has worked directly with many patients at the Alfred Adler Mental Health Clinic, and she has been a member of our treatment staff. We are gratified that her work with our patients is congruent with our own approach to treatment and that the results she has achieved with our patients have been most gratifying.

For these patients the liberating aspects of dance therapy, the relative ease of achieving a positive constructive relation to the therapist, and the stimulation of motivation toward emotional health have all been characteristic of Mrs. Espenak's work.

It is therefore our opinion that her book, based as it is upon both her original and collaborative work in this field, can provide a needed text on the theoretical and applied fundamentals of psychomotor and dance therapy theory. We are sure that our colleagues in the broad field of psychology and mental health will agree that Mrs. Espenak has made a valuable contribution, in her work and in this volume, to all who are concerned with the amelioration of the emotional, social, and physical deficits that impair the ability of so many individuals to enjoy and participate in the positive aspects of life.

ALEXANDRA ADLER

FOREWORD

W HEN I FIRST met Liljan Espenak about twenty years ago, she was a dance therapist. At that time, dance therapy was an entirely new adjunct to the field of mental health. Liljan Espenak was one of the five pioneers, each working in her own particular environment without knowledge of each other, until in 1965 communication was established and the American Dance Therapy Association was established. Marian Chase was the most famous of these, who first brought dance therapy to the medical profession at St. Elizabeth Hospital in Washington and proved that dance was an effective way to reach the mentally ill and to bring them out of their shells.

Movement is one of the most basic forms of self-expression. Through such self-expression, particularly in the form of dance, a person strengthens the sense of self. Dance movements are especially suited for this purpose because they contain a large involuntary component stemming from the rhythmic element in dance. Rhythm is a bodily function. Through dancing, one becomes identified with the body. This identification is the foundation for the growth and development of the ego.

The idea of using the body directly in the therapeutic process to heal emotional illness was introduced and developed by Wilhelm Reich in Norway in the years 1936 and 1939. I was a student of Reich's from 1940 to to 1953 and in analysis with him from 1942 to 1945. The therapeutic approach used by Reich at that time was called "character-analytic vegetotherapy." This approach involved a determination of a patient's character from the expression of his body, that is, from its form and movements. It also involved special techniques for influencing personality through direct work with the body. Bioenergetic analysis, which I developed in 1954, deepened and extended this approach.

Liljan Espenak was attracted to Bioenergetic analysis when I described it to her at our first meeting. She became a member of the Institute for Bioenergetic Analysis and attended the clinical seminars of the Institute for many years. She has a good understanding of the language of the body and of the energetic factors which determine behavior. Thus she brings to dance therapy and to this book a depth of perception about body movement which is quite unique. Her ideas about how movement can be studied and used to enhance personality growth should be very valuable to anyone interested in dance therapy or any other form of therapy.

ALEXANDER LOWEN, M.D.

PREFACE

In undertaking the preparation of an explanatory and instructive work in a discipline such as dance therapy, one first discovers that it is almost impossible to treat the subject in the manner of a formal text. Dance is an art form, and even when it is used in a clinical setting as a form of scientifically based therapeutic intervention, dance remains a fluid, individualized expression of both therapist and patient alike. Consequently, one fails dismally in attempting to set up structures—directive guidelines for the transmission of techniques to others who wish to specialize in the field of dance therapy—for the blunt reason that a certain sensitivity to body "language" must indeed be part of the personality of the therapist. In a certain sense, the would-be therapist must also be a dancer, and by that I mean that the individual must feel, as dancers do, that in the movements, gestures, and stance of the body all emotions can be experienced, expressed, and perceived. It is not a question of sophistication in dance skills as much as it is a question of recognition of the liberating power of the dance, expressed even in its most rudimentary and awkward movements by the emerging personality of the patient.

It is quite possible that my work as a therapist and my outlook as a dancer may well have resulted in offering the reader what appears to be a pastiche of *science and poetry. The dance therapist functions in two worlds,* and this dual approach characterizes the nature of this book.

We live in an almost totally verbalized society, with constant acceleration toward that direction by the media. There is virtually no airspace left for silence and no lifespace for the individual whose trauma lies below the level of talk. It is perhaps difficult, in a culture that believes that everything can be solved by discussion, to understand the plight of those who cannot effectively express their emotions in the popular manner, whether from psychological or physical impairment. It is even more difficult to understand that there are those who cannot *experience* their emotions with intellectual recognition as most of us do and in this sense who remain blocked to their own feelings.

For patients with problems such as these, the world of gesture, posture, and movement provides a medium in which they can not only express themselves to others, more importantly they can learn in this world *to express to the self*—to bring buried, distorted, or immobilized emotions to the surface through the catharsis of movement. *In a certain sense, dance therapy can be considered a primitive technique, and it is precisely the "natural man," the primitive in our patients, that we are trying to release.* The sensitivity, then, of the therapist to this particular form of human expression is a prime prerequisite for effective work; dance therapy *is* a communication therapy, although non-verbal, and it is vital to the interaction that both therapist and patient can "speak" and understand the same language—the language of the body in all its motor manifestations. By the term "dance," I refer to an entire constellation of physical expression, whether the single movement may be a threatening gesture of anger or a joyous jump, just as we would regard the stylized postures of certain oriental configurations as "dance" and as we would regard certain forms of absolute stillness as "dance." Insofar as movement, posture, or gesture represents communication—to the self, to the therapist, or to the group—that movement is "dance," and encouraging and stimulating the patient to use and enjoy that method of communication is one of the major objectives in dance therapy. If a patient who comes to us with a fearful, timorous, sideways walk can reach the point where he can run freely and swiftly across the floor, that is both "dance" and "therapy," because the patient has abandoned certain rigidities, has overcome certain fears, and is beginning to utilize and enjoy the natural spontaneity of his body.

It should be clear from this brief discussion of "dance" as therapy that the development of dancing skills is not a clinical objective. It may be a delightful outcome of the integrative work, but it is by no means a goal. *The goal, if there is one overriding goal, is the restoration of damaged aspects of the*

personality, either through dance therapy as primary intervention technique or as ancillary treatment in support of any of
several forms of psychotherapy or other behavior modification
techniques.

This very basic explanation is necessary because of the dearth
of literature on dance therapy and its relative recency in terms of
established research and practice. While there is considerable
literature and major practice now associated with psychomotor
therapy, as reviewed in detail in Chapter 1, there is very little
reference work to be found on dance therapy as a professional
specialization. This book represents a pioneer effort in the field
of psychomotor study that has been without published guidelines up to this point. The material offered here is derived from
years of professional work in the field, reinforced by study and
research in psychomotor theory.

Many of the procedures introduced in this work evolved from
work with emotionally disturbed adults and children, released
mental hospital patients in aftercare, and the mentally retarded.
Some of the procedures in this book are original, such as the
Movement Diagnosis Tests in Chapter 3, the formulation of
treatment techniques in Chapters 4 and 5, the adaptation of group
therapy techniques in Chapter 6, and the various diagrams and
scales used throughout the chapters.

In many ways the problems confronted in years of clinical
experience were original—in terms of psychomotor applications.
It then became necessary to devise original solutions. It is
undoubtedly one of the virtues of pioneering in a professional
field that one is forced by the absence of authoritative references
to be inventive; it was also part of my good fortune that the
absence of professional voices forced me to pay very close attention to the silent communications of my patients.

Perhaps the greatest good fortune of all was the opportunity
to work in this field, first in Europe and then in the United
States, and to form professional relationships with theorists and
clinicians in psychomotor therapy and in related disciplines. For
instance, in my study at the Alfred Adler Institute and later
my activity as a member of the staff at The Alfred Adler Mental
Health Clinic, I have been able to share a focus on verbal and

nonverbal communications. It is my pleasure to acknowledge a very major debt to Dr. Margaret Giannini, who was Director of the Mental Retardation Institute, New York Medical College, Flower and Fifth Avenue Hospitals, New York City, for offering me the opportunity to develop a teaching program based on my work with the mentally retarded. My indebtedness is very great to Dr. Harold Michal-Smith, Professor of Pediatrics and Psychiatry, Associate Director, Mental Retardation Institute, New York Medical College, now the Program Director of University Affiliated Facilities, Mental Retardation Institute, New York Medical College at Valhalla, New York, since my ten years of teaching at that Institute as an Assistant Professor and Coordinator of Postgraduate Course in Psychomotor and Dance Therapy was made possible by his interest, support, guidance, and encouragement. His advice and experience was invaluable in drawing up the training program and in retaining its high quality with additions of timely lectures and field trips, thus giving the course its high rating as a training opportunity in dance therapy. He also supported and sustained my enthusiasm when the going was rough.

Of major impact in the development of my theoretical and practical applications in psychomotor therapy is Dr. Alexander Lowen, who is indeed the outstanding contemporary psychiatrist in this growing field. My membership at the Institute of Bioenergetic Analysis and my attendance at Dr. Lowen's seminars and case presentations provided a very necessary enrichment to my own work experience.

In another area, that of dance itself, I express my gratitude to Don Farnworth, whose special approach to teaching dance for professionals provided me with many inspirations for my own techniques with patients, and to Isidor Schapiro, who helped me with typing the original manuscript. I also most gratefully acknowledge the editorial assistance of Mrs. Mildred Navaretta, who showed the most unusual understanding of this very new material, and Mrs. Naomi Rosen, who with genuine interest and expertise typed and perfected the final manuscript.

The most sacred debt of all is to our precursors for the development of knowledge regarding the interaction of psyche and soma, particularly those whose inspired research opened up new frontiers of possibility for patients who were not accessible to verbal forms of psychotherapy.

Let us say that dance therapy as just one of the methods for nonverbal intervention may not be considered necessarily more effective than music therapy or art or poetry, all of which serve well as ancillary techniques and as liberating agents for creative forces. There are, however, aspects that make dance therapy unique as a resource for nonverbal treatment. First, creative movement is a function of our innate biological rhythms and is thus closer to natural human expression than any other art form; second, dance alone among the arts engages the total physical being, and in so doing, makes an art object of the self. Thus, in dance one creates no product really. One simply recreates the self, as self and as object, in the continual, harmonious integration and reintegration of body and mind.

CONTENTS

If you're going to write in books, use a pencil

DANCE THERAPY

CHAPTER 1

DANCE THERAPY: THE OVERVIEW

THE THEORETICAL PERSPECTIVE

T HE BASIC VIEW underlying the concept of dance therapy is that the expressive aspects of a personality, in its gestures, movements, and postures, are a function of the individual totality: the intellectual, emotional, unconscious, and somatic totality. Given this totality, it is therefore theoretically possible to provide effective therapeutic intervention at any level of these behavioral modes, due to the phenomenon of their interaction.

At the most obvious level, we can perceive, for example, in the expression and movements of a bereaved person the physical manifestation of intense grief; the emotion felt is non-verbally expressed by the body. Similarly, we can perceive the expression of joy through the appropriate gestures and movements; we observe distinctions in posture between depressed and nondepressed individuals. We see, in short, highly differentiated types and qualities of postures, gestures, and movements in relation to the respective individual psychic environments. At a more complex level, we recognize as accepted formulations in contemporary behavioral science the interaction of conscious and unconscious states, muscular functions, visceral functions, nervous system functions, glandular functions—in effect, all of the systems of the living being as an expression of the totality of that being. We accept that change in any one or more of the inner systems will produce some degree of change upon mental and emotional states.

The field of psychosomatic medicine, for example, is based on the awareness of the identity of many somatic processes with psychological phenomena. Implied in these identifications is the concept that the living being expresses himself in inner and outer bodily manifestations more clearly than in words. In posture, in pose, in mannerism, in attitude, in gesture, in movement, and in breathing, the individual communicates with an eloquence that transcends his verbalizations and that surpasses his own perceptions of his inner state. We also expect, simply as observers of human nature and not as professionals in this field, that changes in this inner state, whether spontaneous or a result of therapeutic intervention, will be manifested in some corresponding change in his visible affect. We would expect that a depressed person, whose physical aspect and movements are slow, heavy, and sagging, will, upon effective intervention in the form of chemotherapy, psychoanalysis, or other appropriate therapies, resume or exhibit more positive expressive behaviors as a result of the diminution of the depression. However, how does this work the other way around? That is, will therapy that is directed toward his muscular and gestural affect also produce change in his mental and emotional states? Alexander Lowen,[1] in discussing the theoretical basis for his work in Bioenergetic Analysis and Therapy, put the question this way:

> Can one change the character of an individual without some change in the body structure and in its functional motility? Conversely, if one can change the structure and improve its motility can we not effectuate these changes in temperament which the patient demands?
>
> In his emotional expression, the individual is a unity. It is not the mind which becomes angry nor the body which strikes. It is the individual who expresses himself. So we study how a specific individual expresses himself, what is the range of his emotions and what are his limits. It is a study of the motility of the organism for the emotion is based on an ability "to move out".

Our focus on the physical dynamics of character structure and on the language of the body is the result of major research in psychiatry, psychology, and the related behavioral sciences, starting perhaps with the prophetic insights of Charles Darwin,[2] who a century ago stated:

> The movements of expression in the face and body . . . serve as the first means of communication between the mother and her infant. . . . The movements of expression give vividness and energy to our spoken words. They reveal the thoughts and intentions of others more truly than do words, which may be falsified. . . . The

free expression by outward signs of an emotion intensifies it. . . .
He who gives way to violent gestures will increase his rage; he who
does not control the signs of fear will experience fear in a greater
degree; and he who remains passive when overwhelmed with grief
loses his best chance of recovering elasticity of mind.

As long as one continues to maintain a concept of separation,
a duality in the body-mind relationship, it is correspondingly
difficult to comprehend the unity of the organism, as evi-
denced and described by Lowen or by Darwin, each at their
place in the historical spectrum. However, once we are able to
view the human being as he actually is and actually functions,
that is, as a dynamic interaction rather than as a set of parts,
it then becomes possible to see the relation of outward movement
to inner movement and to accept the reciprocity of both, in either
direction.

This mutuality of engagement among physical and psychic
systems is the basic concept of psychokinetic theory. The following statement made by Paul Schilder,[3] another of the pioneers
in this field, is indicative of the psychokinetic theory:

There is so close an interaction between the muscular sequence
(involved in all expressive movements) and psychic attitude that not
only does the psychic attitude connect up with the muscular states,
but also every sequence of tensions and relaxations provokes a
specific attitude. When there is a specific motor sequence, it
changes the inner situation and attitude and even provokes a
phantasy situation which fits the muscular sequence.

Common experience serves to demonstrate the validity of this
statement; for example, in an activity such as dancing, the
movements to rhythm and music often "provoke" the flow of
fantasies that are both appropriate to and derivative of the
particular muscular sequence. In free running we have another
example of a certain kind of exhilaration that stimulates changes
in mood and in fantasy. Experiences of this sort are all part of
ordinary human reactions and interactions with various forms of
muscular sequence.

Freud himself, although primarily intellectual, and verbal
in his approach to the psyche, was not insensitive to the possibilities of inducing, inciting, or stimulating emotions by nonverbal means. Several of his comments and letters to colleagues

indicate his interest in this; in one of his letters to W. Fliess in 1899, Freud[4] mentioned that "from time to time I visualize a second part of the method of treatment; provoking patients' feelings as well as their ideas, as if that were quite indispensable."

The history of psychoanalysis does indicate a number of experiments, trends, and concepts toward the release of feelings through an approach to the soma. One of the important thinkers in this regard was Wilhelm Reich, who regardless of some disagreement with his later work was primarily responsible for enlarging the scope of the psychoanalytic technique to include the physical expression of the patient. Another major innovator along these lines was Ferenczi, with his "activity" technique, or "analysis from below". Lowen[1] describes Ferenczi's concept of "activity" as follows:

> It is in line with Ferenczi's concept of "activity" to ask a patient to breathe easily and naturally during the therapeutic procedure. Of course, like all activity procedures, the application is individual; it depends on the particular patient and his situation. It constitutes, however, a basic procedure. In addition, other suggestions for activity or restraint are used, all of which are designed to bring the patient into contact with or awareness of a lack of motility or a muscular rigidity. The dissolution of the rigidity is obtained through the patient's conscious control of the muscular tension and of the emotional impulse blocked by the spastic condition. Movement and expression are the tools of all analytic procedures and these are supplemented where necessary by direct work upon the muscular rigidity.
>
> It is important to recognize the power inherent in these procedures. In this technique, one deals not only with the "derivatives of the unconscious" but with the unconscious mechanism of repression itself. In this way it is possible to bring affects to consciousness with an intensity which is impossible on the verbal level.

This passage serves, in its clarity and conviction, to provide the constructs upon which the field of psychomotor therapy is based and in which dance is conceived as ancillary therapy. The postulates of psychomotor therapy indicate that psychic change can and does occur in relation to change in somatic affect. This premise is primarily a conceptual shift, not in the area of presumptively localizing the cause or source of psychic disturbance in the motoric dimension but in establishing a broader view of the nature of interactive phenomena as it occurs among the component functions of totality. As in other forms of intervention that attempt to contribute to the authenticity of self-perspective, dance seeks to bring the individual to a greater degree of unification in awareness of self through its therapeutic techniques.

THE THERAPEUTIC PERSPECTIVE

In the theoretical construct for the effectiveness of dance therapy, there are a number of factors that are integral to the concept of dance as a basic human activity and that are particularly appropriate for use as therapeutic tools. The most significant of these factors, from a therapeutic point of view, are the following:

1. The stimulation and release of feelings through body movements and gestures.
2. The release of communication and contact through non-verbal activity.
3. The reduction of anxiety through the noncritical aspects of the therapeutic setting and through the suspension of self experienced in dance.
4. The experiencing of physical and emotional joy through the impact of auditory stimuli (rhythm) together with freedom of movement.
5. The use of the innate human response to rhythm in order to generate both individual movement and participation in simultaneity with others.

There are, of course, considerable therapeutic ramifications of the five basic considerations thus far presented, which are discussed in full in their relation to the application of techniques, but for the purposes of this overview, a brief elaboration is now devoted to these five major components in the therapeutic framework of the dance.

Stimulation and Release of Feelings

It is hardly necessary to indicate how, in normally healthy individuals, the charge of emotion is released in body movement. The swift and joyous skip of children on their way to play, the dragging steps of a person in grief, the forceful step of the angry person moving toward confrontation—these are all the everyday observations of feelings expressed in movement. In the last analysis, every movement and every motor action of the body depend upon and express some change or indication of feeling and purpose, influencing the expenditure of energy and the timing of the action. The free release of the dynamic feeling will organically create its own individual form and organize itself, through the various body systems, in its required time and required space.

In the same context, the inhibition or reduction of dynamic feelings, whether in joy or grief, in anger, or in pain, reduces the thrust of energy discharge and reduces the expression of the personality in time and space. The spontaneity is deadened and results in a blocking or a distortion of the original feeling and its original energy. With this also occurs a fragmentation of identity, in the sense that the wholeness of the personality has not been expressed.

Each individual organization in time and space is unique to a personality; the manner of handling the expression in time and space is part of the life profile. For example, the apparently simple act of breathing is an expression of that profile. The emotional significance of respiration is clear when one thinks of the child holding his breath, of the person panting in fear, of the quick inhalations in surprise, of the percussive breathing in sobbing. The use that an individual makes of the expressive functions in respiratory activity is an indication of certain aspects of his personality, and as such, it becomes one of the most important tools in therapy. The ability of the therapist to sense the breathing action, to interpret its tempo and emotional significance, and to offer appropriate opportunities for improved release in improvisational activity is the beginning of the psychophysical approach to therapy.

The same principle applies to the therapist's awareness of all body movement—its deficits, its restraints, its inappropriatenesses—and the disturbances that are indicated by various immobilizations and blockings of the charge of emotional energy.

The opportunity for change, through the dynamism of the

dance, is directed primarily at the release of feelings hitherto blocked in both verbal and motoric expression.

Communication and Contact

Communication is a major goal in dance therapy. Since all communication, whether verbal or gestural, is directed toward someone, the dance has the aim, among its other aims, of making contact with another human being, a group of human beings, or even a god. Szasz[5] describes this matter of contact as the object-seeking and relationship-maintaining function of language, and he makes this interesting observation.

> This viewpoint is especially relevant to the intepretation of such things as the dance, music, religious ritual, and the representative arts.
>
> In all of these, one person can enter into a very significant relationship with another by means of a non-discursive sign system. Using a pharmaceutical analogy, it is as if the language—dance, art, etc., were the vehicle in which the active ingredient—human contact—is suspended and contained.

The sign language of movement then becomes human contact. This contact is easier for many patients to establish with the therapist and with each other—easier that is, than the reliance on direct verbalization. At another level of contact, the dance offers a methodology for the patient to communicate with himself; movements permit the expression of feelings about which the patient may have no conscious cognition or that he cannot express to himself in verbalized thought.

Reduction of Anxiety

The concept of psychological "safety" is very much a part of the therapeutic setting in dance. Maslow[6] refers to this concept of safety as follows:

> Here we can learn important lessons from the therapy situation— the creative educational situation—I believe also creative dance. Here where the situation is set up variously as permissive, admiring, praising, accepting, safe, gratifying, reassuring, supporting, unthreatening . . . non-comparing . . . then it becomes possible for

him (the patient) to work out and express all sorts of lesser delights, e.g., hostility, neurotic dependency.

Once this is sufficiently catharted he then tends spontaneously to go to other delights which outsiders perceive to be "higher" or growthward, e.g., love, creativeness, and which he himself will prefer to the previous delights, once he has experienced them both.

It is also possible that the therapeutic agent in dance is similar to the therapeutic function of dreams, in the sense that both are created by the spontaneous overflow of powerful feelings, both generate an archaic content, both produce a reprieve from reality, an occasional suspension of the inner trial and the inner disbelief. In dance therapy the patient shares in a process of recreation—the vaporous, undefined and troubled feelings are drawn into a form and movement that are conscious and functional—longer and longer intervals of well-being are experienced as the effects of "reprieve," the suspension of the conscious self, are consistently experienced.

Experience of Joy

Dance in itself provides a sensory-oriented, as well as a motor experience, a combined impact of the two sensations. The first is derived from the auditory stimuli with response to rhythm, the second from the feeling evoked by the freedom of movement with its release of inner tensions. It produces a quality of spontaneous abandonment, a surge of natural spirit, a sensation of joy in being alive. This experience, half sensual, half spiritual, is therapeutic in itself as shown in history all over the world.

This joy in the dance, even in the more moderate experience of normal people, serves almost as an antidepressant and as an awakener of a feeling of new possibilities of life, with a capability of living in psychophysical harmony within oneself.

The cumulative effect of these experiences of joy is thus not merely a stimulation of pleasure, but it becomes a motivational aspect of therapy, a stimulation of the desire to recapture this experience again and more fully.

Dance therapy is in fact one, if not the only one, of the psychotherapeutic approaches that can counterbalance some of the pain of dealing with unconscious conflict with the experience of physically oriented release and joy. This element is central to its effectiveness.

Response to Rhythm

Perhaps the most profound catalyst in dance therapy is rhythm. Clinically, we are aware that each individual has a personal pattern, in terms of his outward and inward rhythms, but rhythm is an integral component of human response behavior. The birth process itself is a rhythm of contraction and relaxation. There are tribes that use magic dances to bring on and to accelerate the rhythmic contractions of the mother's womb. The response of infants to the soothing qualities of being rocked or swayed is another obvious, universal example of the effect of rhythm upon the organism.

In dancing one surrenders to the rhythm of music. It is possible to feel an archaic, almost cosmic response to the fall and swell of the beat, as the body yields to the rhythmic occurrence. The moment there is the repetitive sound of rhythm, there appears a possibility for response and sharing; we see the young child in this spontaneous response, clapping his hands and swaying in time with the cadence. Meerloo,[7] has made some pertinent comments in regard to rhythm:

> Future study will have to direct greater attention to the analysis of these phenomena. The compulsive patient, for instance, cannot step out of his own rhythms and obsessive repetitions without displaying enormous anxiety. Psychodynamically, it is known that the compulsion to repeat rhythmically is often used as a defense against the shock of new adaptations . . . certain rhythms may interfere with existing defensive rhythms and thereby open new roads of communication and new adaptation.
>
> Music and dance, the rhythmic intercommunications of man, were once the first forms of magic medicine. Indeed, the common regression to a cluster of interactive movements gives delight and catharsis and revitalizes us.
>
> . . . rhythm in any form expresses many feelings that were repressed formerly . . . rhythm is the integration of chaotic inner and outer events into one's own "musical" experience . . . rhythm can completely revolutionize our body system.

Rhythm also generates a participatory, as well as a self-expressive behavior—participatory in the social sense of joining and sharing a simultaneity of experience with others and participatory in the sense of sensory and emotional relatedness to other stimuli, such as the pattern of instrumental sound. The sensual pleasure of rhythm in dance is a therapeutic experience in itself; moreover, the response to rhythm provides another pleasurable dimension in the freedom of improvisation.

A rite and a magic spell, a joy, an offering, a language in gestures, a welcoming and a farewell, an interpretation of myth and a glorification, a celebration of life—all this is the dance in its multiform aspects, its rhythmic and expressive movements, its flowing from and to the psyche, the mind and body in reciprocal unity.

The universal role of rhythm and dance is an integral part of man's heritage, and its role as activator, catalyst, and outlet is part of virtually every culture from the primitive expressions of tribal man to the extremely formal and disciplined movements of the dance as art form in the sophisticated societies. *The historical role of rhythm and dance, in terms of its relatedness to emotional and psychic needs, is an important frame of reference for dance therapy.* As part of this overview, then, the theoretical and therapeutic formulations so far expressed in regard to dance as activity can be enriched by a brief review of the dance in the historic sequence of the cultural perspective.

THE CULTURAL PERSPECTIVE

The use of rhythm making to induce certain body states, from trance to frenzy, to release emotions into kinetically felt experiences, to provoke emotions through the motor experience, to communicate emotions to the audience, and to stimulate emotions in the audience are part of the tribal history of man. Kurt Sachs,[8] writing in *World History of the Dance* states:

> The dance is the mother of the arts.
> Music and poetry exist in time; painting and architecture in space, but the dance lives at once in time and space. The creator and the thing created, the artist and the work are still one and the same thing. Rhythmical patterns of movement, the plastic sense of space . . . these things man creates in his own body in the dance before

he uses substance and stone and words to give expression to his inner experiences.

. . . the dance breaks down the distinctions of body and soul, of abandoned expression, of the emotions and controlled behavior, of social life and the expression of isolation, of play, religion and battle . . . in the ecstacy of the dance, man bridges the chasm between this and the other world, to the realm of demons, spirits and God. The dance has become a sacrificial rite, a charm, a prayer, and a prophetic vision. It commands and dispels the forces of nature, heals the sick, links the dead to the chain of their descendents. It assures sustenance, luck in the chase, victory in battle, it blesses the field and the tribe.

Although not specifically developed from the psychotherapeutic point of view, the implication of these comments have decided relevance to the integrative functions of dance as *therapy*. Sachs thus indirectly sets the ambience for therapy itself in terms of the healings of body, mind, and spirit through the release of emotions in religious or tribal ceremony, the living out in body movement of both common life and crisis situations.

Historically, the dance has served, for both dancers and audience, as a representation or a direct expression of the major emotional states, encompassing the great many nuances, the shades and degrees of intensity within the major emotional categories of *anger, joy fear,* and *calm.* As we move into the direct relationships of postures, movements, and gestures to the spectrum of emotional states through the technical developments in later chapters, the precise reciprocity of feeling and muscular affect will be accordingly elaborated, but for the purposes of this overview we will now confine the discussion to the concept of catharsis as expressed by dance in the cultural perspective.

ANGER: *In primitive man the war dances indicate the transformation of fear and anxiety into courage and aggression, the coming-of-age dances are reflective of anticipation and joy.* In the ecstatic dances we see a catharsis, an abandonment to the affirmation of life. In the ritualistic expressions of tribal experiences we see dance used as a communal expression along with individual identification with that shared experience, reinforcing a sense of belonging and security. Voodoo dance ceremonies in Haiti, for example, provide observations on religious expression as mode of catharsis for universal, that is, existential anxiety.

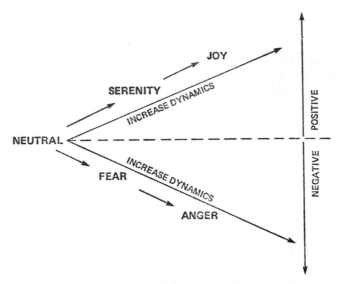

Figure 1-1.   Increase of dynamics.   Four emotions.

The voodoo priests first prepare the "floor pattern," designs drawn on cornmeal, which was previously scattered on the ground. These intricate floor patterns are dedicated to whichever specific god the tribe has selected for supplication. While the priests prepare, the members of the tribe begin to throb to participation by the sound of the constant drumming and monotonous chanting and clapping. Offerings are made with formal repetitive movements. The group will continue the series of their own spontaneous primitive movements until one or another of the participants reaches the experience of being "beside himself," that is, the sensation of being possessed. As a representative of the tribal emotion, this individual will step into the center of the ring of tribesmen, and with squirming, snakelike movements, he will indicate the incarnation of the god—the snake god in this example. Crawling, wriggling, and shaking in complete abandon, a dance of complete submission to the god, a tribal release or a communal catharsis occurs, in this transmission of human responsibility into the hands of the god, seeking the protection of the god.

Albert Schweizer,[9] in his reports of the Leopard Man in

the east coast regions of Africa, describes war preparations through the dance, where the dancers strive for identification with the various wild beasts in the environment. They dance until they feel possessed by the animals that they are impersonating. Losing their own sense of individual ego along with its attendant fears and anxieties, they then literally, in the guise of the respective animals into which they have surrendered the human personality, abandon the dance to pursue and fall upon the enemy in the manner of the beasts.

In both of these examples, the ritualistic dance in honor of the snake god or the tribal dance to simulate the courage and ferocity of the wild animals, we see the phenomenon of tribal identification with images or organisms considered to be powerful. We see the use of repetitive sound and rhythm constantly accelerating with the movements of the dancers until a genuine immanence or transcendence is achieved—in effect, a cathartic release of the self.

There are, of course, innumerable examples in the literature of research into primitive dance to demonstrate primitive man's use of the dance to induce other states of consciousness through reaching forms of trance, hypnotic states, orgiastic states, ecstatic states.

One of the best known of the primitive ecstatic dances is the Bulgarian Fire Dance, where worshippers leap into the embers of a giant bonfire and dance in the ashes to a wild beat of drums and bagpipes. This frenzy increases until a trance is reached. In this semiconscious state, the person spontaneously verbalizes myth and prophecy.

Dances of this ecstatic type are also undertaken to cure "insanity" in tribal members; certain cultures in Bohemia and Poland have the rites of the St. Vitus Dance, which reach a similar pitch of semiconscious trance. The "sitting dance" of Bali is another example of reaching the hypnotic state through swaying back and forth continuously to a monotonous drumming.

Primitive dances were obviously thus utilized in a variety of ritualistic, improvised, and spontaneous movements for mental and emotional transcendence. They were also used for a sense of communion and relatedness to the group. In therapy the basic elements of the primitive dance are effective for providing initial release of life energy and anger, without the necessity for formal training of body movements. The percussive quality of the instrumentation and the repetitive rhythmic movements in individual expression produce a spontaneous, nonverbal involvement by the patient in the feeling and in the activity.

JOY: *As many cultural forms of expression became more sophisticated in the developmental context of earlier societies, new considerations were evolved in regard to the exercise of restraint, choice of movements, and related aspects of shape, form, content.* The power, wild energy, and spontaneous abandon of the primitive dances became slowly transformed, along with other cultural changes, into disciplined forms, such as the ritual dances in Crete, in Greece, in Egypt, and in Persia. The cultivated expression of great calm, of tranquillity for example, is described by Sappho of Lesbos: "Thus, in olden times, did the Cretan woman dance to the tune of music, with tender feet, around the charming altar, treading the soft flowers of the lawn." As another example of the evolvement toward control, Egyptian dance became a disciplined performance of trained dancers conducted in honor of the various gods and goddesses. It was highly controlled and formal, communicating a grave and measured concept to the audience.

In the classic Greek culture, the purpose of the dance was to achieve and communicate emotional balance and aesthetic form. The thematic content persisted, as with primitive man, indeed as in all dance, but it became controlled and enhanced, stylized by form. In this early Athenian civilization, the dance became an expression of the Greek philosophy, which was oriented toward balance based on a fusion of beauty and health, the idealization of man tempered by moderation and balanced in body and mind, and an embodiment of the soul within, expressed in a harmony of rhythm, form, and movement.

In therapy today, we seek to help the patient find this unity, utilizing certain movements to achieve mental organization through body organization, and to increase the conscious experience of interaction between psyche and soma in terms of a mutuality of balanced engagement, as balance creates joy.

CALM: *The search for a unity of emotional and physical balance, a tranquillity, in effect, of the body/mind unity, takes on a special form in the culture of the East that is a different type of solution through dance movement.* Dances of the East are characterized by whirling movements, monotonous and continuous, following the principle of the unending circle. The circular movement may continue indefinitely without a new impulse, providing a sense of freedom from the bonds of gravity and a feeling of communion with a larger universe. These whirling movements tend to produce an inner tranquillity, and for many of the dancers who adhere to this form, the dance becomes a vehicle for deeper voyages into the self. The best known example of this are the Whirling Dervishes, who continuously turn their bodies until they reach cosmic or religious experiences that lead them to a renewal of spirit.

Another famous example of the dance evoking states of calm and tranquillity is the Hawaiian dances, with the monotonous circling of hips and hands. Westerners who perform this easy-flowing dance and genuinely respond to the sway of the rhythm can be observed to undergo certain changes, such as the relaxation of facial tensions and body constrictions different from the habitual field of consciousness.

FEAR: *One of the major functions of dance, historically in the elimination of fear, has been to provide identification with entities that appear to be more powerful than the self,* to suspend egotistical functions with their accompanying distress, as exemplified earlier in the descriptions of primitive dance identifications with wild animals, in the war dances, or in identification with one of the tribal gods, as indicated by the religious, ceremonial dances. In the original imitation of animals and nature by primitive man, it was believed that the dance in reality affected the animals and gods—that by donning the mask or imitating the movements the dancers acquired their qualities—the courage of the lion, the ferocity of the tiger, and so on. This dance of identification, or the suspension of self, has appeared as part of virtually every culture. This is seen in the gold masks of the Egyptian dancers, the dragons of the Indian and Chinese dancers, the Japanese Noh masks. The various cultures have all recognized this type of transcendence of self, not only as the need for identification with a greater power but also as a technique for the expression of inner powers that are blocked by the mechanisms of the repressions normally associated with acculturation, even in a primitive form. The mask, as used in both primitive and sophisticated dance, also provides "safety" for the expression of feelings and attitudes that are either emotionally or culturally repressed.

In our own Western culture, the strongest representation of the mask was the commedia dell'arte, which emerged in the Middle Ages in Europe. The mask dances of this period are probably the best examples known to us of the use of the mask as a "safe" outlet for many forms of expression. In the historical context, the use of the mask emerged as a reaction to the religious prohibitions of the church during the eighth to tenth centuries, particularly those directed against the pleasures of the body and the expression of physical or sensual enjoyment in the dance. These prohibitions were severely repressive but could not, nevertheless, erase the need for expressive movement as emotional release. Since the church could not abolish the practice, it incorporated it into its acceptance of the carnival celebrations. Paul Nettl,[10] a major music historian, writes the following in his book, *Story of Dance Music*:

> Originally the name of the festival was Carrus Navalis, the Ship on Wheels, which carried the leader of the ancient chorus and dances, Dionysus, during the rites for the god of fertility. The name itself had to adopt a new etymological explanation and became "Carne Vale", meaning "Farewell, precious flesh", as it was brought into religious relationship in the fast during Lent.

The improvisations during the carnival processions became the traditional entertainment for the people on their feast days. Improvisations gave vent to the full imagination and feeling, uninhibited and released from the standards of behavior imposed upon them in their daily life. The mask took on traditional meanings, and as the severity of the church lessened, the emergence of the use of mask and mime as an art form, as theatre, occurred. With the enjoyment of freedom behind the mask, the dancers were thus able to depict with increasing talent and sophistication the satire, the ribaldry, the wit, and all of the feelings and attitudes the culture did not permit for expression in other forms. The mask, in effect—*and it is in this context that we see the tremendous application for dance therapy*—took the burden of responsibility for all repressed or unacceptable feelings, offering its wearer a place to hide and yet to be fully expressive without fear of punishment. In this manner and through the language of movement, dancers participated in a "confessional," a cleansing, and a release.

The therapeutic possibilities of the mask are considerable; the patient's reactions to masks provide valuable information in terms of preferences for certain masks, the rejection of certain masks, and so on. Basically, the mask functions as a tool for the suspension of the conventional self, as a vehicle for identification, and as a safety device for the outlet of repressed emotions, attitudes, and desires.

In the developmental context of dance history, the use of the masks ultimately became formalized, just as the dances of primitive man became formalized through its translation by the successive classic societies. In Japan, for example, Kabuki became an offshoot of Noh and now coexists with it.

For the ultimate display of organization and control of dance movement as an art form in contemporary society, one looks to the classical ballet of the West and to Kabuki in the East as the epitome of perfection in form and discipline. Again, coexisting with the control and integration of highly disciplined dance movements are the modes of freedom, spontaneity, and improvisation as expressed in popular dance movements today.

In a certain sense, dance therapy seeks to reproduce, working with patients in the psychological environment, the evolution of the history of dance, providing within a clinical setting the opportunity for the acting out of fears and anxieties through the archaic, primitive movements of the tribal man. It then seeks to develop the fragmentary experiences into more integrated expressions by offering the mask as an intermittent refuge from the oppression of the conscious self; and by seeking once again to integrate the emotions and attitudes into conscious expression and coordinated controls.

THE TECHNICAL PERSPECTIVE

In all forms of gesture, movement, and posture that are manifested in ordinary daily life, we see the expression of the personality, and we perceive through our personal sensitivity (particularly so with training) the constellation of emotions, blocked or free.

The haste with which an angry mother runs after the naughty child is a different expression from the dynamics of her walk, when, hand in hand, mother and child walk together toward some pleasurable event. We contrast the movements of people walking behind a coffin, slow and burdened with grief, with the joyous running and skipping of children when school is out. We observe an individual waiting on a train platform for the arrival of a lover. The expression of the waiting individual is impatient; he is pacing back and forth, standing for a moment, looking at the clock. The train approaches, and the body dynamics change. The head rises, the body stretches and breaks into a running pace along the platform. When the loved one is sighted, the run accelerates, and the arms are held out. This is, in effect, a dance—a dance in its release of dynamic feeling, in the creating of a sequence of movements in time and space. A different type of "dance" sequence is expressed if the meeting on the train platform involves waiting for a business associate to arrive. The individual would stand in a corner, perhaps, reading a newspaper. As the train approaches, he will slowly fold his paper, slowly walk out on the platform, meeting and greeting the arrival with a courteous handshake. It is another "dance" entirely, but it follows the same principles of feeling and attitude as dynamic energy, formulating its organic expression through motor movement in time and space. Daily life for all of us consists of these expressive sequences.

Looking at these sequences in the technical perspective, we see the dynamism of emotions expressed in body movement. In our first example of the mother running after the child, we see the temper aroused, thus increasing the energy charge of her body-mind unity and accelerating her movements. Her pace and forward progression in forcefully running after the child clearly expresses two related emotions—*anger and aggression.*

In the next example, where child and mother are strolling hand in hand, we see that the dynamics have been defused, the mother has returned to her original serenity, influencing the energy output and tempo. Now she exhibits a light and even gait. Her movements are indicative of *calm, tranquillity.*

In the funeral scene, the person laden with grief will have little dynamic drive to expend on progression; the weight of his feelings will slow him up; he walks without spring or forward drive. His gait, his demeanor, his posture are indicative of *grief, fear.*

At the other end of the emotional spectrum, we see the dynamics of happy anticipation as the children rush from the discipline of school out into the street. The spirited movements of skipping and running clearly express *gladness, joy.*

Thus, in these simple everyday experiences, we see the dynamics of the four major emotions expressed: anger/aggression, calm/tranquillity, grief/fear/anxiety, gladness/joy.

Every motor action of the body relates to some change in feeling or interest, influencing expenditure of energy and the timing of the action. The free release of the feeling *will organically create its own form and organize itself in its required time.* In these examples it has been assumed that the various individuals thus exemplified are secure enough in their own respective identities to be free in their expressions and are able to release their feelings (their dynamic energy) in spontaneous and appropriate movement.

But, where an individual suffers from a number of blockages, ambivalences, inner confusions, and restraints, the various psychological mechanisms involved will impair the free flow of the emotional dynamism. For example, some children in the vicissitudes of their growth find that holding their breath makes them more insensitive to unpleasant sensations and feelings. They pull in their bellies and immobilize their diaphragms to reduce anxiety; they deaden their bodies to avoid the feeling of pain or anxiety. In this defense, they avoid pain, but they also deaden themselves to *all feeling,* including happiness and joy.

By the reduction of dynamic feelings, the dynamic energy is also reduced, with consequent diminishing of the expression of personality. The spontaneity is lost; the self-awareness and the self-identity are impaired and incomplete.

Although the examples given are universal, the actual organization of a personality is unique to that personality. Each individual has his own inherent personal dynamism, his own inner and outer rhythms, and these rhythms express a personality that is both total and unique. The individual's personality experiences change as he moves through life, but that change follows his own unique pattern, it represents at any given time the total of his physical/psychological/social heritage plus his unique interpretation of his own life history.

The ability of the therapist to sense the unique rhythm of the personal dynamics, to appreciate the influence of the expressed tempo and its emotional origins, and to offer appropriate opportunities for the dynamic release of that tempo in improvisational activity is the beginning of psychomotor intervention, as realized in dance therapy. Experience of one's own rhythms is an experience of self-feeling, an experience of integration of movement and emotion. To offer the patient an opportunity to arrive at this experience, the realization of self, is one of the major goals of dance therapy.

In the technical construct, the therapist learns how to interpret the total motor expression of the patient, how to relate personal movement to personal feeling, and most importantly, how to reach the feeling through specific opportunities for specific experiences in movement. *The physical phenomena provokes the occurrence of the emotion.* This is the foundation of the therapy.

In the ensuing chapters we will deal with the technical applications of dance therapy, demonstrating the relatedness of movement to feeling and of specific movements to specific feelings. We will review the diagnostic tools of dance therapy, the methodology of assessment, a view of the current functions of interaction in the total personality of the new patient, and a view of the progress made in terms of first releasing and then integrating the dynamics of this interaction.

The fundamental goal is to restore, to the maximum degree possible within the context of a given personality, the lost unity of the living systems. To accomplish this objective, the therapist requires not only training in concept and in technique but also the capacity to bring his or her own unity to the therapeutic situation.

REFERENCES

1. Lowen, Alexander: *The Language of the Body.* New York, Macmillan, 1971.
2. Darwin, Charles: *The Expression of Emotion in Man and Animals.* London, John Murray, 1945.
3. Schilder, Paul: *The Image and Appearance of the Human Body.* New York, Intl Univs Pr, 1950.
4. Freud, Siegmund: *The Origin of Psychoanalysis.* Letters to Wilhelm Fliess, New York, Basic Books, Inc., 1954.
5. Szasz, Thomas S.: *The Myth of Mental Illness.* New York, Har-Row, 1974.
6. Maslow, Abraham: *Toward a Psychology of Being.* New York, D Van Nostrand, 1968.
7. Meerloo, Abraham Mauritz: *The Dance.* New York, Chilton, 1960.
8. Sachs, Curt: *World History of the Dance.* Seven Arts Publisher, Norton & Co., Inc., New York, 1952.
9. Schweizer, Albert: *Philosophy of Civilization.* London, Macmillan, 1949.
10. Nettl, Paul: *Story of Dance Music.* New York, Philos Lib, 1947.

CHAPTER 2

PSYCHOMOTOR THERAPY

IN THE SITUATION referred to in Chapter 1 of the lover waiting for the beloved at the train station, we observe his difficulty in standing still. He wishes to remain composed, but the intensity of his excitement makes it impossible to contain the feeling within his body . . . the pressure of his emotion presses his body outward into space, forcing him to pace back and forth. As the train approaches, his mental focus on the awaited object now seeks its own physical expression; his body straightens, and his head lifts in anticipation. He glimpses the beloved in the distance as the people swing out of the stopped train. All need for further restraint vanishes, and the free flow of his feelings stream outward into space with his forward run. As he closes the distance between them, he opens and lifts his arms, making his total forward body-thrust complete, in one flowing line. We have, in this one example, the interaction of psyche, mind, and body—harmonious, integrated—in the dance of life.

In psychomotor therapy we are concerned with the interruption of the fluidity of interaction in this unity of psyche, mind, and body as manifested in psychological and physical behaviors and with the application of theory and technique for restoration to the maximum degree possible of this natural fluidity. The therapeutic intervention required for this task takes its direction from a number of significant constructs, which follow.

BODY IMAGE

The terms body image, body concept, body schema, body perception, body ego, and body experience are often used interchangeably and often without preestablished definition. The meaning of these terms often depends upon what one is trying

24

to describe or explain. The wide range of phenomena indicated by these terms overlap in nature as well as in semantics; when we try to isolate certain observations in specific conceptual terms, the definitions become somewhat arbitrary. Nevertheless, we must assign consistent referents to significant terms and, in doing so, attempt to avoid both contradiction and redundancy.

The term "body image," as it will be used in this discussion, is a psychological construct; it is used to describe the visible affect of the inner personal view of the body. The term "body experience" comprises the sum of the factors of body image and body movements, as viewed by the self and as viewed by the observer; it encompasses the reactions of the self and of others as these factors become incorporated into the personal experience of inner self and outer world.

Body image is one of the major aspects of the total self-image. It constitutes the personal psychological/visual interpretation that each of us maintains in regard to the personal physical body and its affect. One may for example, "feel" that one is beautiful but that either no one or everyone recognizes this to be so. One may feel that one is ugly but that this is an inner secret which no one else can know—in other words, the belief that the body does not betray the psychic secrets. In these simplified concepts the idea of body image is not limited to the self-concept but includes the inner idea of how one appears to others. For example, a schizophrenic may feel such self-loathing that he considers his body to be dangerous to the touch of others. Another psychotic fantasy may be that one's body does not exist; therefore, the person thinks he is invisible to others.

Body image, then, is a subjective view of one's own physical body and of the reactions of the self and others to that manifestation. Body image is therefore susceptible to disorders in self-perception and to accompanying disturbances in both the conscious and unconscious aspects of personality. The degree of disturbance may range from the bizarre, compulsive rituals of the psychotic to the constricted and self-conscious postures of the frightened, timid person. At either end of the psychic spectrum, the disturbance of the body image development will be reflected in the physical aspect and movements of the body.

The formative knowledge about one's body is developed, biologically, through cortical organization of data derived from internal and external stimuli that are initiated by the self and significant others. This sensory information is eventually organized to the level at which the child differentiates his body from those of others—humans, animals, objects. Concurrently, the child is also experiencing the attitudes that he later internalizes, which become part of his individual psychic, emotional, cognitive, and intellectual constellation.

As the child grows and enters peer group relationships, he acquires additional data, which are derived from comparison and interaction with others. The body image first developed in the family setting is then confirmed, negated, or modified by other developmental experiences as the child moves into and through adolescence. During the strong emotional, social, and sexual pressures of this period, he again reevaluates, reaffirms or negates, exaggerates or diminishes, substitutes or recomposes his self-view in response to the social criteria of his milieu and the events, occurrences, triumphs, and defeats as he subjectively experiences and interprets them. There are, then, a *series*, of body images at this time, which are transient, experimental, fluid, layered, split or integrated. Eventually these images are developed into a relatively fixed adult body image.

Obviously, the transitions to this point represent a complex process; the amount and variety of input is vast, the personal vulnerability of the human is equally great, and the need to develop coping strategies to regulate this interactive dynamic is a matter of psychic survival. Insufficient experience, defective experience, traumatic experience—all can occur at any point along the line or may be occurring sequentially to reinforce previous experiences. Thus, the development of a "healthy mind in a healthy body" reasonably related to objective reality and to the genuine potential of the individual is, for many, a perilous passage.

Apart from or in addition to the obvious distortion of body image and movement in situations where organic impairment exists, there are the limitless and unquantifiable existential factors to which each of us is uniquely exposed. The parental attitudes are, of course, a major example. Parental eccentricities, norms, values, and attitudes toward the body and/or its various parts are translated into psychic idiom and egotized in the psychological development of the child. Some of this parental emphasis may be of a type that is detrimental to the growth of an adequate body image. For example, attitudes of shame or disgust may lead to corollary attitudes in the self and to consequent mechanisms of denial, displacement, alienation, and so on. Where disapproval or lack of affection for the child's physical self occurs, the child may perceive his own body as unworthy of his or anyone else's libidinal investment. This may lead to devaluation of his total self-esteem.

The central problems that occur as a result of or concomitant with distortions in body image occur at three levels of the personality: (1) defects in the sense of identity, (2) misconceptions in self-perception and in the interpretation of the attitudes and reactions of others, (3) relative immobilizations, rigidities, and tensions in parts of the body or in an overall diminished body tone. The specific mechanisms involved are unique to the individual, but the intensive research undertaken by significant professionals in this field of inquiry provide some generalized understanding.

Historically, the research into body image began with Henry Head,[1] whose orientation was physiological and primarily concerned with the organization of stimuli and perception. His work continued in a direct line to Paul Schilder,[2] who in effect placed the physiology in a psychological perspective with this statement: "When we perceive or imagine an object, we do not act merely as a perceptive apparatus; there is always a personality that experiences the perception." In this book Schilder directly employs psychoanalytic concepts to explain the role of the body image in such conditions as neurasthenia, hypochondriasis, depersonalization, pathogenic pain, and hysteria. Schilder thus moved the thinking on body schemata and their automatic functioning to a new theoretical level with reliance on the construct of the ego and endowed the development of body image and self-perception with the unique voluntary processes, conscious and unconscious, of the individual. Lowen[3] in *Betrayal of the Body* carries the psychoanalytic construct further with his studies of the schizoid and schizophrenic personalities, in which he describes the relationship between body image, ego, and personality as follows:

> The ego depends for its sense of identity upon the perception of the body. If the body is charged and responsive, its pleasure functions will be strong and meaningful, and the ego will identify with the body. In this case, the ego image will be "grounded" in the body image. Where the body is "unalive" pleasure becomes impossible and the ego disassociates itself from the body. The ego image becomes exaggerated to compensate for the inadequate body image.

The assumption that the ego is capable of functioning and influencing behavior relatively independently of the body continues to be reflected in recent research and in contemporary therapies, such as biofeedback, and in existential psychiatry. Szasz,[4] for example, speaks of "messages from the body to the ego" and states in reference to his analysis of the experience of pain that the body "denotes whatever is so recognized by the ego." Shontz[5] in his work on personality refers to a significant study of body images as follows:

> Fisher and Cleveland (1951) characterized the body as a "unique projection screen for patterns of attitudes." They identified the body image not as a spatial-geometric reconstruction of the person's body but as a representation "formed of these projected attitudes." In fact, they went so far as to say that we have almost taken the 'body' out of 'body image' by postulating that the body image does not really mirror the actual properties of the body surface, but that it is rather a representation of attitudes and expectancy systems which have been projected onto the body periphery."

These "attitude and expectancy systems" appear to be components of the internal body image, but they also affect the interpretations of the body images of others. Schilder[2] very strongly emphasized that the body images of separate individuals engage in exchange and interaction, stating that

> There is continuous interchange between parts of our own body image and the body images of others. There is projection and appersonizations. But in addition the whole body image of others can be taken in (identification) or our own body image can be pushed out as a whole . . . the body images of others and their

parts can be integrated completely with our own body image and can form a unit or they can be simply added to our own body image and form a sum.

These observations on identification are relevant to some of the discussion on the history of the dance in Chapter 1, where the animal dances of primitive man precisely recapitulate the identification with the strength and ferocity of specific wild beasts; it is not a mimicry of but an identification with the animal. As to the comment on "pushing the body out," this affect (depersonalization) has been described by Lowen, Laing, and others in the case of schizophrenic patients, who have expressed feelings that they are disembodied, without bodies, separated from their bodies.

In addition to the bulk of work that has been and is being done on the body image disorientations of the psychotic, there is intensive study of body image distortions or disturbances in the area of personality research. Personality-oriented research is characterized by the premise that the body either determines or serves as medium for the expression of individual traits. These traits and characteristics are regarded as significant indicators of important processes in personality development. Apart from the clinical observations in this area, the validity of these assumptions is confirmed at the everyday level of perception that we, as ordinary lay observers, bring to the interpersonal scene. We conduct informal personality research based on body observations in our daily life and in our daily language.

We say that an individual who is "down to earth" or has "his feet on the ground" is one who has achieved a certain control over his life. Conversely, we describe an individual lacking self-assertion as "tiptoeing around" or "dragging his feet" or "pussyfooting around." The popular term "hung-up" illustrates almost literally the state of insecurity; the feet appear to be, indeed, off the ground. If legs are strong and sturdy, the person is seen as independent, "He can stand his ground." If he is dependent, he is "weak kneed," "hasn't got a leg to stand on," is "down on his knees." We notice that a back "arches in pride" or bends over in humiliation; it is "spineless" as an indication of weakness in the character. A person "bends over backwards" when seen as willing to conciliate or stands "stiff as a ramrod" when inflexible. Numerous degrees of forward and backward bends and other changes in posture will produce equally varied interpretations of personality or mood. The shoulders "shoulder the burden." They can be drawn "up to the ears" in fear or anxiety, as if protecting from a blow. A "chip on the shoulder" is dignity offended; to shrug indicates that a given responsibility is abandoned.

We "reach out" to the world with our arms. When we cross our arms in front of the chest, we are refusing contact. We "receive with open arms," or we hold others "at arm's length." We can hold out our hands for the handshake and yet retain the arm close to the body in a reluctant, ungiving, or untrusting way. We "lend a helping hand" or we turn a hand up and palm out to say "stop." We associate emotions with the chest: sorrow is the "pain in the heart"; "breast-beating" indicates guilt; surprise "takes the breath away"; we "hold our breath" to express suspense or avoid pain; the chest is touched in various ways for a reinforcement of feeling. All of these gestures generate a number of popular interpretations.

These various aphorisms indicate the ordinary approach to the reading of "body language," and they indicate the manner in which the individual conveys, through his body stance and movement, the communications of feelings and attitudes to others.

From a clinical point of view, however, our concern is directed primarily at those constellations of physical aspect which indicate varying degrees of disruption in body-ego harmony. The fundamental focus is, of course, on the total affect of the individual, but certain body behavior syndromes, in regard to posture, movement, and muscular tension, fall into recognizable patterns that can be considered pathways to the clinical perceptions of personality disturbance. We shall consider here some of the major manifestations that we see in therapeutic practice.

HEAD AND SHOULDERS: The carriage of the head is expressive of the way the individual feels about his intellectual position vis-à-vis the world of others and about his ability to control his emotions. The way the chin is held is indicative of the interpersonal stance: aggressive refusal, truculent distrust, determination, obstinacy are indicated by the degree of uptilt. The head thrown back in defiance is the most common example of the outthrust chin. However, the head may also be straining upwards, the neck elongated, in a striving for spirituality or, in a more bizzare manner, to express a desire to be free of the body, to deny that the body exists.

There is often a lack of alignment between the head and the rest of the body and a rigidity of shoulders and neck, expressing an attitude of disdain and withdrawal, as if one were, as Lowen[3] says, "above the bodily pleasures of life." When the head commands primarily, with nonacceptance or denial of body strivings, we find the "cut off" forward tension, accompanied by body immobility. Bending to the side, in effect keeping the head tilted, the evasive quality inherent in sideways movement, becomes evident, which indicates indecision and distrust.

The downcast head blocks out the world. The visual and emotional focus is the self. The introspective forward bend of the head denies all options for new views and ideas. The head needs to come up, so to speak, for "air."

Rigidity of the head and shoulders, one of the most common aspects of the schizoid personality, often gives the arms the appearance of being suspended in their sockets, more like appendages than as integral components of the body.

CHEST REGION: The constricted, cramped chest so frequently observed in the postures of withdrawal and depression is of particular concern because of the interference with breathing. In therapy, the new experience of "opening up" the chest through the programmed breathing and shoulder swings designed for correction has often the most dramatic effect. The anxiety during the beginning of the routines can be observed, followed by the equally discernible shock of realization that an inner constriction is lifting and that free movement is flowing. With continued therapeutic experience, the vise of the chest stance changes to a posture of relaxed freedom, permitting the adjustment in the alignment of the spinal column and with it, the deep breathing that is essential to body and psychic health.

THE "DIVIDED" BODY: There are a number of other distortions, which are characteristics of both the neurotic and schizoid personalities. The upper half of the body may be muscularly underdeveloped, with a tight thorax held in a somewhat collapsed position. This posture, of course, affects the breathing and limits it. There is often constriction at the waist, giving the impression of a "split" in the body between the upper and lower half. The patient often unconsciously identifies the upper half with his ego, his self-control, his intellect; the lower half represents the rejected sexuality, the "lower" mechanisms of the body. The pelvic structure indicates this psychological affect.

THE HIPS AND THE PELVIC GIRDLE: The inhibitions are usually very obvious in their physical effects on posture and mobility of the sacrum and hip joint. Fear or guilt feelings about sexuality often retract the pelvis, overexaggerating the lumbar curve and creating the swayback; the buttocks can be so tense in the effort of closing all body openings that the pelvis is tilted forward and under. Some maintain a constant tension in their thigh muscles by pressing them close together, unconsciously still behaving "properly" as they were told. Whatever different causes to which the tensions can be attributed and whatever changes they have caused, the goal must be to reestablish the full mobility of the pelvis, allowing it to carry out the involuntary function of co-ordinating the lower limbs with the spine and head in its daily life of activities and to function in freedom and harmony in sexuality. In the case of obesity, surprising changes can occur after a program of relaxation of sacrum and thighs instead of the energy-consuming violent exercises mainly used for losing weight. The pelvis must be allowed to swing freely, performing its circular movement at every step, supported by the legs over which it can sway like a hammock between two trees.

These examples indicate the relationship between personality and body behavior. More specifically, they indicate some of the more obvious ways in which the self-view, with its accumulated repressions, inhibitions, fears, longings and aims, shapes a perception of one's body and how that perception in turn influences the development and perpetuation of observable and definable body aspects. For significant changes to occur in the personality and in the emotional and functional behavior relative to the world, changes must occur in body image. In appropriate situations, this effort can be undertaken through the verbal techniques of psychoanalysis or other intellectually focused therapies, which seek to reach the unconscious fundamentally through the mind or through a nonverbal approach to the unconscious through the body, which constitutes psychomotor therapy. In the psychomotor view, the dynamics of body, mind, and psyche are not those of separate entities but are one total expression of the individual personality, and they form an interdependent unity for healing.

BODY MOVEMENT

Life—that is, the organism in interaction with the environment—offers its possibilities for survival through movement. This life force is demonstrated at birth in the jerking, random movements of the infant. The only apparatus we possess for the acquisition of data pertinent to survival is the sensory equipment, and this is so linked with the motor systems that sensory impression can be viewed, in terms of function, as the preparation for muscular action. Of course, man has developed inhibitive, selective intellectual capacities over the past 50,000 years or so, which minimize the need to make overt movements responsively to sensory impressions, but the point is that we are alerted and prepared to make them in the appropriate situations through our neuromuscular system.

In a society such as ours in the last decades of the twentieth century, where the emphasis on practical and scientific intellectual performance constitutes a popular religion, it may be salutary to consider that intellect is really a very recent development in man's evolution; therefore, it presents a rather limited section of mankind's total experience. It is not capable, as a function in itself, to set up any communications with reality and can only act upon that data which are supplied to it. The intellect serves basically as an organizing, conserving, and interpreting function. For the raw input of life—that is, experience—for perception in its most potent and profound sense, and for the consequent enrichment of capacities provided by that perception, we must call upon that larger portion of our existence which is supraintellection, paraverbal—discoveries and recognitions of intangibilities which are, in fact, the basis of both science and art.

It is the purpose of all humans to convey their personal perceptions of reality to others; this is the fundamental communal communication, whether it is the croon of the mother to the infant at the breast or the sophisticated commentator broadcasting his analysis of political events. This communication of perception is not confined to an Einstein's perception of the universe nor to a Proustian conception of society. We are all, in terms of personality, what we perceive. Therefore, what we call psychosis, neurosis, aberrant behavior, and so on is fundamentally, highly individualized distortions of perception in relation to what more of us view as reality.

What we are trying to do in psychomotor therapy is to encourage expression of these highly individualized perceptions in response to inner impulse and memory, and to tap the unconscious, submerged, repressed material that for certain kinds of individuals has no satisfying channels for release other than the most basic of all communication channels, that is, movement. The use of dance techniques, as dance therapy, is a heightening of movement beyond the boundaries of ordinary motor activity. Dance therapy utilizes the inherent power of movement to open a channel of expression and communication for the patient through rhythms, music, improvisation, and other stimulation techniques. Its focus is the movement evolved from the patient's perception of his body and its relation to time, to space, to floor, to walls, and to others. Its subject matter is the raw material of the patient's personal experience. Its form is the shaping and organizing of this raw material to render it intelligible to the patient and to others.

Kinesiology is the science of movement, the knowledge of how the body moves and how the parts function and relate. The dance therapist, of course, not only must be versed in the kinesthetics of the body, which may have been acquired by formal dance training or by the "doing" in dance training but must also have a trained understanding of anatomy, that is, of the parts and their natural functions in movement.

Our model is the ideal body—that is, one that works perfectly in terms of the natural functions of posture and movement. For example, the diagnosis tests that are discussed in a later chapter are based on the degree of departure from these ideal characteristics. The first focus in the study of movement—from a slight stir to total body involvement—is not on *what* the patient does but rather on *how* he moves to do it. With certain patients who are for a variety of reasons significantly immobilized, our first task is to get them to move, not simply by verbal instruction to do so, which may be ineffective, but by a range of stimulation techniques directly addressed to the body. Thus, movement itself is the starting focus in the dance application of psychomotor therapy, for it is through movement that the individual expresses his life force and its associated individual characteristics.

When we look at movement in the dance context, that movement takes on two additional dimensions. One is expression, and the other is communication. These expressive and communicative movements, however, do not take place in a physical or social vacuum; they take place in a definite space, in relation to measurable time. They occur, on one hand, in an identifiable social and cultural milieu, but they also participate in universally recognized gestures and other dynamics related to common human emotions and thoughts. For the organization of these universal aspects of movement in space and time we are indebted to Rudolph von Laban[6] whose theoretical formulations, as of the midtwentieth century, were the first comprehensive efforts to develop an objective method for the study of movement expression and communication behavior in dance.

Laban postulated that there is a correlation between oriented forms of movement and a certain harmonious arrangement of their sequences in space. To illustrate the specific relationship of body movement to space, Laban developed the concept of the "dimensional cross." For example, in a simplified version if one makes movements with the arms from the center of the body outward to the space around, then simple dimensional directions of height, breadth, and depth occur. Six points of orientation are then immediately established: height, depth, right, left, back, forward. Movements toward each of these points offer their own particular expression. Reaching up, for example, expresses a feeling of longing or aspiration; reaching down is sadder, more contemplative. Moving the arms out from the body side indicates an awareness of others; an arm movement across the body brings about a closing movement, shutting others out. Backward movements tend to be timorous, retreating, forward movements are advancing, extending, assertive.

Of course, Laban is describing conscious, volitional movements of trained dancers, whereas in therapy we would see these untrained movements as individual dynamics involuntarily expressed in forms—a dynamics-forms concept rather than an effort-shape one. However, the meanings conveyed would be identical—the discharge of pleasurable tensions creates a movement forward and upward. Fear, sorrow, and disappointment would be visible in movements backwards and downwards. In moving sideways, the individual expresses avoidance, the desire to escape.

The use of space in movements also indicates psychological or emotional states. If an individual has no strong sense of boundaries, he will tend to be a larger user of space or intrude into the space of others. The opposite feelings—unworthiness, inadequacy—can be recognized by the sidling movement or the use of as little space as possible.

The important point regarding Laban is that what is formally established as conveying emotional states by formal dance movements is, in fact, the natural expression of untrained individuals making movements in space. *It is precisely this universality of movement language that gives dance, as art or as therapy, its enormous powers of communication.*

Laban's contribution centers upon the formalization of certain basic postulates: that all movements are executed in definite directions in space; that the greater variety of conceivable movements relates to three fundamental dimensions, i.e. high-low (height), right-left (width), front-back (depth). Most of the freely executed movements follow these three dimensions and therefore their diagonal supplements.

Laban carried out the supplements and variations with

technical precision, using for directional diagramming the geometrical figure of the icosahedron, a perfectly symmetrical polyhedron providing both spherical and cube dimensions. The dancer, in actual movement, does conform to this figure in that he is able to execute spherical movements and that he is essentially limited by the three-dimensional symmetry of space represented by the cube, that, is height, width, and depth. In effect, the Laban icosahedron with its twelve points surrounded by twenty triangular places is a technical movement scale that can be used by the dancer to regulate the force (dynamic) elements and the emotional elements of each movement.

Laban influenced a number of famous dancers in Europe, such as Mary Wigman, who in turn created her own sphere of influence upon the development of modern dance. Mary Wigman was perhaps the most influential of the followers, since she brought a high degree of both creative and training ability to Laban's organization of space and movement dynamics. A part of Wigman's creativity training consisted of "exercises" in relaxing intellectual focus and permitting emotions to come to the fore, an approach which later found its relevance to the techniques of dance therapy.

Other exponents of the new approaches to dance movement were Isadora Duncan, as a purely personal exponent, and in America, Ruth St. Denis and Ted Shawn, who founded the Denishawn School, with an approach described as "giving freedom to form and form to freedom." Three important dancers came out of this school, each with respective dance concepts: Doris Humphrey, Charles Weidman, and Martha Graham, all of whom formed respective schools and spheres of influence.

Modern dance, however, is not the only source. Physical techniques, where applicable in specific patient situations, are also derived from relaxation techniques by Alexander and Jacobson, swing techniques are from Bode and Medau (Germany), Dalcroze methods (Switzerland) are used in relation to rhythm; yoga is used for its technical focus on tranquillity; dervish turns are employed for trance; psychodrama is used for its expression of roles in interpersonal situations; and even games, gymnastics, and folk dance are used for particular adaptation for the mentally retarded or other types of patients who are inaccessible to more sophisticated techniques.

All of these various sources, and significant new approaches as they arise, are integrated with a psychological approach to develop the dance approach to psychomotor therapy.

PSYCHOMOTOR THERAPY

We have indicated how certain psychological constructs, such as those of body image development and its effect upon physical behaviors, have provided a formal basis for one aspect of psychomotor therapy; we have also indicated how the organization of the expressive and communicative aspects of movement, in terms of its universality of applications in time and space, form another aspect of this therapy. Binding the two together is the understanding of unconscious dynamics, as formulated by significant conceptualizations in psychology and psychiatry. In this context the major influence is derived from the Adlerian concept of treating the triune existence of the individual: (1) the *emotion* being the motivating force; (2) the *mind* organizing the action; and (3) the *body* performing it. The salient concepts derived from Adlerian theory are the following: (1) aggression drive, (2) social feeling, (3) inferiority feelings (and related organ inferiority), (4) life-style (early recollections, first memory). This theory offers itself, almost naturally in its linking of organic functioning to mind and body, as a useful point of departure for relating psychological thinking with bodily function and especially expressive movement, i.e. dance.

While Adlerian psychology and its theoretical model have been a major influence on my psychological techniques of dance therapy, psychomotor theory is also based on a number of powerful theoretical and research formulations in biology, sociology, and psychiatry, as previously reviewed in detail in Chapter 1. We thus have in psychomotor theory, and in its practical expression in the form of dance therapy, a blending of significant resources—psychological, physiological, and dance technique orientations—whose practical application is discussed in detail in the ensuing chapters.

REFERENCES

1. Head, Henry in Allport, G. W., and Vernon, P. E.: *Studies in Expressive Movement*. New York, Macmillan, 1933.
2. Schilder, Paul: *The Image and Appearance of the Human Body*. New York, Intl Univs Pr, 1950.
3. Lowen, Alexander: *Betrayal of the Body*. New York, Collier Macmillan, 1967.
4. Szasz, Thomas W.: *The Manufacture of Madness*. New York, Har-Row, 1970.
5. Shontz, Franklin C.: *Research Methods in Personality*. New York, ACC, 1965 (for reference to Fisher and Cleveland study). (For direct reference, see Fisher, S., and Cleveland, S. E.: *Body Change and Personality*. Princeton, N.J., D. Van Nostrand, 1958.)
6. Laban, Rudolph von: *Mastery of Movement*, 3rd ed. Boston, Plays, 1971.

CHAPTER 3

DIAGNOSIS AND EVALUATION

BEFORE A REVIEW of the specific procedures is presented, there are a number of considerations to be undertaken in regard to the concepts upon which diagnosis and evaluation are based.

APPROPRIATENESS OF DANCE THERAPY

When dance therapy is conducted at a clinic or mental hospital, it takes its therapeutic role as one of the many disciplines in the overall clinical team. As a member of the staff, the dance therapist participates in the periodical discussions of patients and makes recommendations where they are indicated. There may be instances where a nonverbal approach is needed for regressed patients or where a sublimation is needed for aggression, or a buildup of a patient's self-image would be helpful in altering his negative self-attitudes. In these and other areas where our combined physical-psychological approach might be effective, a program of dance therapy is thus instituted to pursue these goals. In such a setting dance therapy would then be a designated part of the total therapeutic management of an individual patient.

Similarly, in private practice the patient may be referred to the dance therapist by the psychologist or psychiatrist or by a clinic. Dance therapy may also be recommended by the referral source as a primary psychotherapeutic technique or as a supplement to other forms of ongoing treatment. Movement —the way one moves, gestures, and postures—is a form of behavior, and insofar as that behavior is erratic, bizarre, constricted, or abnormal in relation to the normal neuromuscular structure of an individual, our therapy is designed to alter it. The ultimate objective is through such alteration to reach and to ameliorate *alternate to talking therapy*

the disorders of the inner state, the emotional perceptions that produce the visible somatic affect. This objective would then be appropriate for emotionally disturbed individuals, for the emotionally impoverished, and for those who through deficiencies in the familial or environmental setting have not enjoyed the normal prerequisites for emotional maturation. Dance therapy would also be appropriate for those with relatively normal movement behaviors but whose shyness or intense self-consciousness or low self-esteem tends to restrict their freedom of the body as a pleasurable instrument of life. Dance therapy would also be indicated for those individuals who, for a variety of reasons other than physical or sensory disability, are inarticulate, who cannot verbalize their feelings and thoughts, and who thus suffer from a high degree of frustration in communications and in relationships.

There is another appropriate population who is similarly handicapped through problems arising from physical or intellectual limitations: those who are mildly mentally retarded, those who are mildly brain damaged, those who are nonviolent autistic and schizophrenic patients, and those who have mild sensory system deficits (speech, vision, or hearing impairment). These deficits are often accompanied by moderate personality disturbances, which are reflected in body behavior.

A considerable amount of work in this field is undertaken with children. It is, of course, an equally effective therapy with teens and adults. The entire field of psychomotor therapy— dance therapy, movement therapy, paraverbal therapy— is relatively new, and the possibilities for application have by no means been fully explored. We may find, as clinical research and experience expand in this field, that there are appropriate applications to the alteration of delinquent and criminal behaviors, addictive behaviors, and so on. Therefore, while we have indicated the various broad dimensions in which dance therapy is presently conducted, the field of additional possibilities for application is by no means circumscribed. There are, however, certain behaviors where this procedure is contraindicated.

CONTRAINDICATIONS

Obviously, dance therapy is a technique that, although it emphasizes spontaneity and freedom of movement, stresses coordination and control of movement relative to respective patient needs. Therefore, the very seriously handicappd cannot effectively participate due to relatively severe degrees of physical impairment. To do so would be counterproductive, in terms of the disappointment and serious frustrations that would result. Again, considering the predominantly stimulating character of dance movement, hyperactive children or adults with strong trends toward acting out their inner violence are not considered appropriate for this therapy, except where strong emphasis is placed on relaxation or monotone movements. The therapy is also contraindicated for the exhibitionistic or voyeuristic patient, who might use the physical aspects of the therapy to reinforce the neurosis. This outcome might well be unavoidable; therefore, other nonverbal therapies, such as music therapy, would not only be more effective but would produce more rapid results. Another category that is considered inappropriate is the custodial retarded, for whom some of the major goals of dance therapy—the motivation and capacity for independence—cannot be realized and where participation may develop severe frustration as well as become an obstacle or threat to the care of the patient. There may also be deterrents to participation in certain cases for a variety of medical reasons, arising from the multiple-discipline diagnoses of the clinical team.

GENERAL PHYSIOLOGICAL CONSIDERATIONS: Apart from the specialized considerations involved in impairment or ill health, there are some general physiological considerations in regard to the program planning and therapeutic goals for patients. All persons are organically destined due to genetic inheritance or developmental problems to have very specific types of neuromuscular structures. Obviously, some are short, some are tall, some have greater or lesser flexibility of the joints, some possess the capacity to develop greater muscular strength than others, some have greater vulnerability to fatigue than others. It is then equally obvious that it is a basic obligation of the dance therapist to be thoroughly *aware* which *physiological resources are inherent* and which are limited by psychological stress and to adapt the techniques properly to the realistic evaluation of the patient.

Dynamically conceived, the therapy is a process of partly effecting change in the personality by modifying physical states, and this modification involves the stimulation and strengthening of muscles, the conditioning of glands, and, in effect, the modifying of the entire neuromuscular system. Large muscle activity is a direct and simple way to stimulate vital processes. Such movement induces increased flow of blood to the brain, stimulates the metabolic and other chemical processes of life, and generally affects the total physical tonus of the individual. While these changes are physiological, they are viewed in dance therapy as interwoven with psychological change, with improvements in ego states reflected in body states, and with improvements in body states reflected in ego states. Therefore, in this view the differences among patients in terms of physical structure, although they may affect certain levels of physical movement, do not at all impede the effectiveness of therapy. In diagnosis, for example, the procedures are designed to focus on the *dynamics of interaction* between body and mind. For example, we are interested in the drive, the mobilization of energy, behind the patient's movements rather than in his muscular strength per se; we are not as much interested in the skill with which he performs certain movements as we are with his willingness and his persistence in the effort. In short, we are concerned with the behavior characteristics of his movements rather than in any absolute conceptions of grace, prowess, and so on.

The diagnostic tests, then, are designed to give us a picture of the total behavior picture in movement and to provide a base for planning a treatment program that encompasses both physiological and psychological needs as they relate to the ultimate integration of one single entity—the personality. There are certain common denominators of the dynamics of interaction among all patients that are applicable to the diagnostic work in dance therapy, namely, rhythm, tempo, form, and space relations. These dynamics are the material that all patients have available as their contribution to the therapy, along with the capacity to develop emotional interactions with the therapist distinct from that of pupil-teacher relationships. During the years of clinical work, the necessity of developing a system to evaluate the potential of each patient on the basis of the common denominators available to all became fully recognized. The following movement diagnostic tests were developed accordingly and standardized for use in clinical practice.

MOVEMENT DIAGNOSIS TESTS

These tests are grouped into seven basic areas, and they comprise both negative and positive components of personality.

1. Degree of dynamic drive (energy)
2. Control of dynamic drive (rhythm)
3. Coordination (neuromuscular functions)
4. Endurance (toleration of frustration)
5. Physical confidence (courage, reluctance, fear)
6. Body image (self-concept)
7. Emotional state (expressed in improvisation)

Test 1: Degree of Dynamic Drive (Energy)

1. Push a chair
2. Push a table
3. Stand against the wall; push back against it
4. Bend knees, push the floor
5. Bend knees, jump in air.

This simple test will indicate the motivation and energy used in accomplishing a physical task requiring some expenditure of force. In the performance of this task, some may apply their entire body to make sure of total strength from the floor; others may use arms alone and often ineffectively; others may turn and use their backs to push; still others may refuse to exert themselves altogether but look around for someone to help them do it. There is obviously a wide range in degrees of energy and initiative utilized in this simple task, as well as judgment in regard to the efficiency of the energy used. How does the individual handle obstacles to the task? Does he remove an obstacle in the path of the table or chair he is pushing, does he push around it, or does he stand still, blocked by it?

In the wall test does the person really use his strength in pushing, or do these elements, wall or floor, which are immovable, discourage him from anything more than a token exertion? In bending his knees and in pushing against the floor, is there determination in the leg muscle, is there flexibility in the bending? Is the bend extremely difficult, moderately difficult, or perhaps impossible? What about the jump—is it done with bent knee? Is there enough drive to do this, enough willing thrust to get him off the ground? Through these nonverbal demonstrations, the therapist forms the preliminary evaluation of the drive available, in terms of both energy and willingness to utilize energy for the challenges ahead.

Test 2: *Control of Dynamic Drive (Rhythm)*

The dynamics in controlling the drive relate to the sense of time in the same way that the previous test related to the concept of energy. Control and organization of time reveals both the individual's inherent personal rhythm and his ability to respond to a given organization of movement within a time pattern, that is, his ability to "cooperate" with a rhythm pattern, alone or with a partner.

We use three methods for our observation:

1. Control of changes in pace
2. Organization of rhythmic patterns
3. Breathing rhythms

The control of changes in pace, or speed, is measured by a simple exercise of "jogging" in place, starting with standing, increasing dynamics to slowly walking, increasing further to running, eventually becoming a run as fast as is possible for that individual. Once the person has reached the peak of applied energy, he will require a gradual decrease of energy or speed until the end shows a complete standstill again.

By presenting changes in the tempo of the music, we create changes in the pace of the movement and thus observe the capabilities for transition. Does the patient make an instinctive adjustment to the change, or does he hesitate or flounder? Is he uncomfortable in making adaptations to change, can he "cooperate" with the music (or with his partner), or does he either come to a halt or persist in maintaining his previous tempo by disregarding the change? Is he listening and responding only to his own inner rhythms or to the music? Can he give of himself to the external organization?

Throughout the phases of this test, observation of the breathing is an important task for the therapist, since the rhythm of the breathing indicates the emotional equilibrium, and also indicates the instinctive adjustment to energy requirements. Breathing rhythms indicate the degree of emotional stability, and the control of those rhythms are also a technique for acquiring that stability and an awareness of the relationship of breathing to alternating experiences of tension and relaxation. Training in breathing is an important function of dance therapy. This test thus indicates patient problems in this area for treatment planning, along with whatever problems appear in the control and organization of dynamic drives.

Test 3: Coordination (Neuromuscular Functions)

By coordination, we mean the total of emotional, mental, and physical control, an inherent capability of the neuromuscular systems expressed in physical movement. The capacity to develop this totality, however, varies with the developmental experiences of individual life. Through adverse emotional and physical experiences, the natural integration of body systems becomes disturbed, and the potential for coordination is blocked to varying degrees. In testing the capabilities in coordination, we start with a return to the instinctual levels of early walking from the position on all fours and then proceeding with the step-by-step utilization of the muscles involved in erect walking. The test calls for a series of movements:

1. Quadruped walk (see Figure 3-1)
2. Biped walk
3. Return to quadruped walk
4. Movements of the sacrum (see Figures 3-2 A and B)
5. Coordinated movement (see Figures 3-3, 3-4, and 3-5)
6. Sideways walk
7. Arm swings (see Figure 4-6)

Obviously, the patient's problems in coordination will become apparent in performing this test and thus indicate the appropriate techniques for correction so that a normally smooth locomotion can be achieved. In normal locomotion an essential factor is the movement of the sacrum, which performs a small, wheellike motion that allows a smooth and relaxed change of weight from one foot to the other. (Note this sacrum function in Figure 3-3 A and B.) The immobilized trunk, which is so characteristic of many patients with inadequate body image and self-esteem, results in disturbances in locomotion, such as jerkiness or rigidity. The walking movements, therefore, which are observed in this test, offer a natural demonstration of problems in interactions, not only among the physical parts and systems but in the harmony of body and ego.

Test 4: Endurance (Tolerance of Frustration)

In the endurance test we use certain techniques for rating such factors as attention span, capacity for tolerating change, and continuity of effort. The test provides two phases of observation:

1. Repetitions of movements
2. Narrowing and widening of focus

From the measurement of patient performance in the test situation, we are able to evaluate his capacity for prolonged activity, his determination under strain, his concentration upon the task and similarly relevant characteristics of his personality and his current attitudes, all expressed in the area of movement in response to organized stimulation patterns.

Test 5: Physical Confidence (Courage, Reluctance, Fear)

Fear is a major component in inhibiting the free expression of feeling in movement. In the following tests, the movements are so constructed as to diminish patient control of the physical situation and to determine the levels of reactive anxiety or fear. The patient is at all times perfectly secure in reality; what we are seeking is any unreasonable or projected levels of fear or

QUADRUPED PROGRESSION

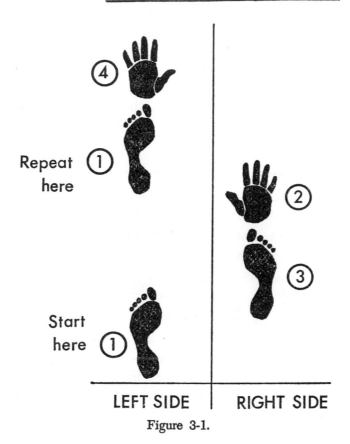

Figure 3-1.

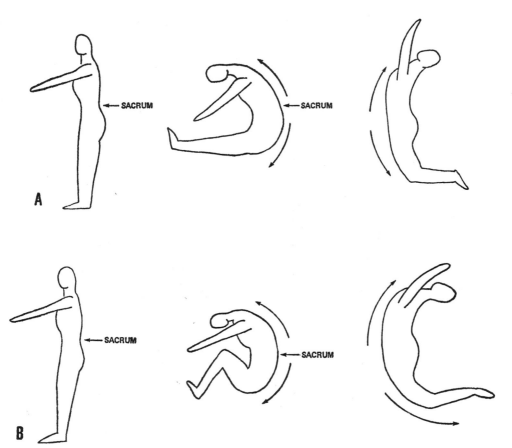

Figure 3-2. **A.** "Shrimp" exercise 1, seen from above, body lying on the floor on the right side. Coordination: movement of the sacrum. Starting from the resting position (left), push out the sacrum, allowing legs to react, which results in a jackknife position (middle). Then push feet and head out from the body as far as they will go, creating an arch (right). Repeat on the left side. **B.** "Shrimp" exercise 2, same view as for A. Push out the sacrum with a thrust, allowing torso and legs to react. This results in a fetal position (middle). Then, push feet and head out from body as far as they will go, creating an arch (right). Repeat on the left side.

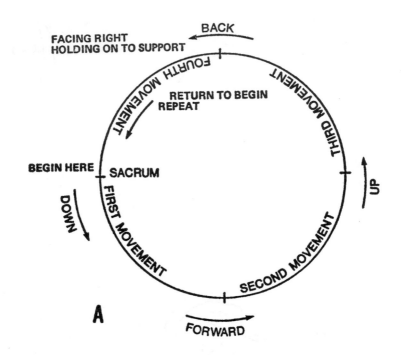

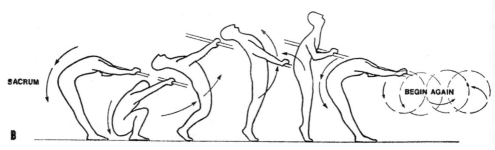

Figure 3-3. **A.** The "wheel" movement of the sacrum without blocks. B. Figure demonstrating the "wheel" movement shown in A.

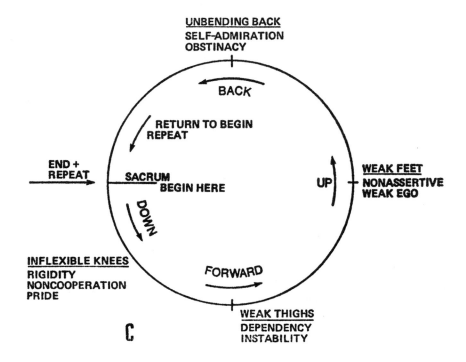

FACING RIGHT
HOLDING ON TO SUPPORT

UNBENDING BACK
SELF-ADMIRATION
OBSTINACY

BACK

RETURN TO BEGIN
REPEAT

END +
REPEAT

SACRUM
BEGIN HERE

DOWN

UP

WEAK FEET
NONASSERTIVE
WEAK EGO

INFLEXIBLE KNEES
RIGIDITY
NONCOOPERATION
PRIDE

FORWARD

WEAK THIGHS
DEPENDENCY
INSTABILITY

C

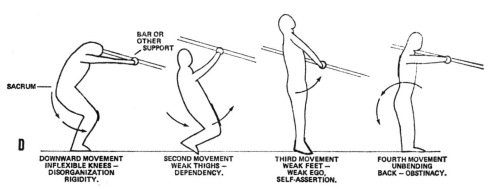

BAR OR
OTHER
SUPPORT

SACRUM

D

DOWNWARD MOVEMENT
INFLEXIBLE KNEES —
DISORGANIZATION
RIGIDITY.

SECOND MOVEMENT
WEAK THIGHS —
DEPENDENCY.

THIRD MOVEMENT
WEAK FEET —
WEAK EGO,
SELF-ASSERTION.

FOURTH MOVEMENT
UNBENDING
BACK — OBSTINACY.

Figure 3-3. C. The diagnostic "wheel" movement of the sacrum with blocks preventing coordination. D. Figure demonstrating the "wheel" movement with blocks appearing in the diagnostic wheel.

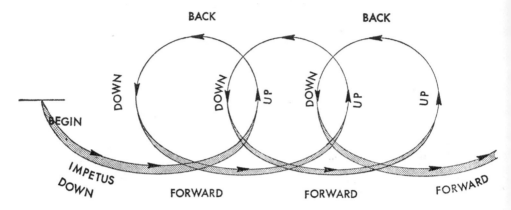

IMPETUS AND CONSEQUENCE IN SUCCESSION

Figure 3-4. Impetus and consequence in succession. Walking movement in a darkened room, with a flashlight on the hip, describing the circular movement of the "wheel."

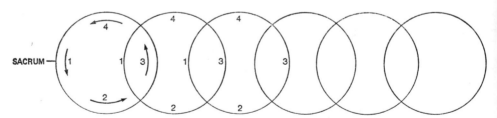

Figure 3-5. Sacrum movement in succession in walking. 1. From sacrum, lift foot in back; move it to front. 2. Transfer weight. 3. Stretch body on front foot. 4. Replace sacrum to free position in back. Repeat sequence.

anxiety upon new physical situations. The tests call for the following movements:

1. Walk backward
   a. Walk backward from wall to wall
   b. Walk a spiral, leaning in to center
2. Roll on floor
   a. Rock back and forth, sitting on floor
   b. Roll backward, legs in air
   c. Roll back and come forward, getting up with crossed legs
   d. Roll backward, touch floor behind head
   e. Somersault forward, backward
3. Falls

Naturally, the therapist must be sensitive to the limits indicated by the patient's behavior and proceed with care where unreasonable fears of falling or of anxiety over limiting the freedom of the head occur. The fears and anxieties, when not appropriate to the physical situations, are closely related to the fears of the patient in his everyday life.

Test 6: Body Image (Self-concept)

This test introduces a simple muscular performance that indicates the ego strength and self-assertive characteristics of the patient in response to the following instructions:

1. Lift on toes
2. Stay on toes
3. Walk on toes
4. Lift arms up
5. Open arms up
6. Lift head
7. Walk forward on toes with open arms and head up

There is no skill required nor is there any demand for muscular strength. Nevertheless, to be able to lift on toes, to stay on them, and to move forward is an indication of the stability of an individual when he is reduced to the smallest base of contact with gravity, his toes. Lifting the arms up—a movement both ordinary and simple—is nevertheless revealing.

Are the arms lifted all the way up, as high as the individual can reach, or are they partially lifted? Are the arms open wide, partially open, or barely opened? Are the palms facing up, out, or down? Are the fingers of the hand closed and stiff or does the hand open also in a free and natural gesture? Does the expression of head movement show ease and confidence in the upward thrust of the body, does the expression of the face indicate the exhilaration normally associated with this upward thrust? Does the patient fall back heavily on his feet, or does he try to prolong the posture and the movement? What feeling does he convey to the therapist as he walks forward, arms up and open, head up, lifted on toes?

Test 7: *Emotional State*

In this final test, we are trying to establish an understanding of the emotional stance of the patient in terms of four basic emotional states: anger, gladness, calmness, or fear. The technique used is dance improvisation by the patient to different kinds of music or verbalized images offered by the therapist. This test, in effect, calls for a spontaneous creative expression in movement in response to specific stimulation; the patient is free to create his own response in movement. By free responsiveness to the music, the patient is sometimes swept along and loses himself in his own improvisation, or he may show resentment and anger in abrupt and jerky movements, or there may be complete resistance to any demonstration of feeling or imagination. Each patient will show a marked personal choice of movement patterns, which will be employed repetitiously. He may use his arms only or his feet only. He may remain in only one place on the floor or move about freely. He may bend his body or hold it rigidly erect. In each case, the therapist will be able to elicit some preliminary manifestations of the emotional climate of the patient in terms of the four basic emotions stated.

We also elicit in this test some idea of spatial relationships, that is, how the patient uses the space around him, minimally or generously. If he bends and moves very close to the ground and his directions into space tend downward, his emotional aspect is obviously quite different than if he leaps, jumps, or seeks to penetrate the space above him. Is he fluctuating among different directions into space, in constant opposition of upward and downward movements? Is there movement in the body center, in the hip girdle, or is he flailing about in space with his arms and legs only, the body remaining immobilized?

The flexibility or the immobilization of the trunk is a significant point for observation, for rigidity of the trunk is indicative of rigidity of the personality—an inhibition or unconscious refusal to experience movement in the very center of life. These initial improvisations are indeed our first view of the patient in responsive movement; it should be clear that he has not been asked literally to "interpret" the music or the verbalized symbol but rather to express whatever energy he wishes to bring to it, whatever movement he feels like making, whatever kind of space he wishes to explore. This test, then, becomes the initial invitation to the release of inner feeling. Obviously, what the patient does not do in his "dance" is as important as what he does. He may be halting, faltering, timidly moving back, virtually standing still, caught in an extreme of self-consciousness, or frozen with fear of movement, or he may move with excessive bravado and assertion, even aggression.

EVALUATION

Evaluation consists of a comparison of performance on the tests to an established standard of harmonious function in movement. It should be understood, of course, that the dance therapist is a professionally trained observer and that referral points in this comparison are technically formulated. The performance on each of these tests is graded; a profile is then developed on the basis of the grades and on the notations of special problems. The clinical picture is summarized, and we thus have the basis for an approach to treatment.

Throughout the test activity we have observed both the physiological and personality aspects of the individual. We have observed his coordination, breathing, poise, placement, and balance, his leg and arm movements, and his shoulder, neck, and torso movements. We have pinpointed areas of reluctance, rigidity, faltering, immobilizations; we have observed both the

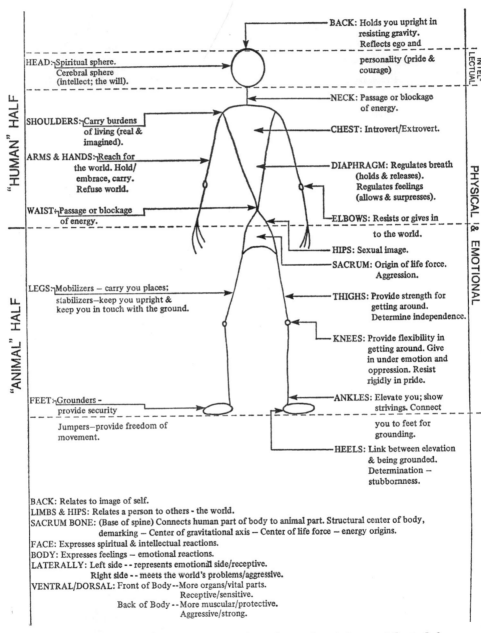

BACK: Holds you upright in resisting gravity. Reflects ego and personality (pride & courage)

HEAD: Spiritual sphere. Cerebral sphere (intellect; the will).

NECK: Passage or blockage of energy.

SHOULDERS: Carry burdens of living (real & imagined).

CHEST: Introvert/Extrovert.

ARMS & HANDS: Reach for the world. Hold/embrace, carry. Refuse world.

DIAPHRAGM: Regulates breath (holds & releases). Regulates feelings (allows & surpresses).

WAIST: Passage or blockage of energy.

ELBOWS: Resists or gives in to the world.

HIPS: Sexual image.

SACRUM: Origin of life force. Aggression.

LEGS: Mobilizers — carry you places; stabilizers—keep you upright & keep you in touch with the ground.

THIGHS: Provide strength for getting around. Determine independence.

KNEES: Provide flexibility in getting around. Give in under emotion and oppression. Resist rigidly in pride.

FEET: Grounders - provide security

ANKLES: Elevate you; show strivings. Connect you to feet for grounding.

Jumpers—provide freedom of movement.

HEELS: Link between elevation & being grounded. Determination — stubbornness.

"HUMAN" HALF / "ANIMAL" HALF

INTELLECTUAL / PHYSICAL I & EMOTIONAL

BACK: Relates to image of self.
LIMBS & HIPS: Relates a person to others - the world.
SACRUM BONE: (Base of spine) Connects human part of body to animal part. Structural center of body, demarking — Center of gravitational axis — Center of life force — energy origins.
FACE: Expresses spiritual & intellectual reactions.
BODY: Expresses feelings — emotional reactions.
LATERALLY: Left side - - represents emotional side/receptive.
          Right side - - meets the world's problems/aggressive.
VENTRAL/DORSAL: Front of Body--More organs/vital parts. Receptive/sensitive.
          Back of Body - - More muscular/protective. Aggressive/strong.

Figure 3-6. An integration of mind, body, and emotions. Adapted from *A New Non-Verbal Approach to Personality Evaluation* by Liljan Espenak.

congruity and incongruity of his approach. We have a view, in short, of the degree of integrity of the body in motion, relative to the physical structure of the individual.

We have learned something of his drive, his tonus, and the degree of his willingness or resistance to participation. We have learned something of his social attitudes as well in terms of his timidity or aggression. We have also been afforded some insight as to his emotional stance. Technically, we have learned something about his spatial behavior; for example, we use three dimensions of space to interpret the emotions of the movements. First, we observe the movements at the middle level of space, which is the normal level of everyday movement, the reality level on which we normally live and normally perform our ordinary tasks. Second, we have the upper level toward which we reach, stretch, raise up the arms, elongate the neck, thrusting up with head or total body or leaping with both feet off the ground. The movement into upper space is an indication of our striving, our aspirations; it is a defiance of gravity, of all that symbolically holds us down. The third level, expressed in crouching, bending, moving close to the earth, symbolizes the longing for security. It also expresses sadness, grief, conflict, and fear. Although technically we use these spatial indications at differing levels as symbolization, the symbols are drawn from the reality of universal human expression of emotions in movement. We owe much to Laban, who was discussed earlier, for his research into the universality of symbolism in spatial movement. We observe the patient communicating these recognized feelings in his choices of space. We also observe three other directions into space, namely, the forward, backward, and sideways movements, that is, the assertive thrust forward, the withdrawing backwards, the avoiding, averting sideways sidle.

PLANNING THE TREATMENT

The approach to treatment is totally individualized. For example, the duration of the treatment session series planned will be based, in good part, on the patient's frustration/tolerance levels, both intellectually and physically. For the mildly mentally retarded patient, where distraction or boredom occurs more easily, a short session, such as twenty minutes, is often more effective. With children, one-half hour is considered ideal, but again, that depends upon the individual child. In the case of neurotic patients in individual therapy, who can sustain acute expressions in that duration, the ideal session could be forty to fifty minutes. Again, for individual therapy, sessions twice or three times a week constitute a productive schedule. In group therapy, one weekly session appears to meet the needs effectively.

In all situations, progress is evaluated at regular intervals by repeating the original test series. If the patient is attending two sessions per week, the tests are repeated every three months. If he is attending one time weekly or less, the test is administered every six months.

The main issue in planning the logistics of treatment is to remember that we are dealing with dynamic emotions and their release. Consequently, we avoid rigidity in rules and attempt to respond, in all cases, to the uniqueness of the individual. The physical program, later described as Phase 1 of the treatment, requires sensitivity to the physical capacity of the patient to respond. Work with older people may be more limited. With teenagers, for example, the full challenge will be offered. In the psychodynamics of the program, which are part of Phase 2 of the treatment, as described in ensuing chapters, the major variable factor is the intelligence level of the patient, regardless of age or physique.

It should be clear that although we describe the program as developed in two phases *both phases are interactive.* The physical approach, in which attention is focused on developing weak, inactive or overemphasized parts of the body, carries over into improvements in the emotional dimension. Similarly, changes in that emotional dimension reflect improvement in the physical area. This concept of interaction is fundamental to the process of dance therapy and its treatment aspects. This will be discussed in the following chapters.

For purposes of testing and evaluation, we use a scoring system for each of the tests relative to individual patient performance, and notations are made relative to each of the tests, as illustrated on the following sample of the Movement Diagnosis

Test Chart. We thus derive a profile of the patient, in addition to the material available from referral input sources, upon which we can plan the techniques to be used in correcting or ameliorating the observed problems and deficits. Our first task, then, is the physical restructuring, which will be described in Chapter 4.

Dance Therapy

<u>MOVEMENT DIAGNOSIS TESTS</u>

NAME_____   DATE OF TESTS _____
ADDRESS _____   AGE_____
_____   REFERRAL _____
TELEPHONE_____
Prev. Exp. with Dance or Exercises: Where:_____
When:_____
Operations or Physical Weaknesses: _____

- -

SCORE
(Ideal) Real

__(25)__   1. <u>Degree of Dynamic Drive:</u>
1. Push chair_____   2. Push table_____
3. (Stand back against wall)   Push wall _____
4. (Bend knees)   Push floor away_____ Jump in air_____

__(15)__   2. <u>Control of Dynamic Drive:</u>
1. Responses to speed _____ 2. Simple Rhythmic patterns _____
3. Relaxation - - rest _____   "Espenak Wheel"
· Obstruction Where?

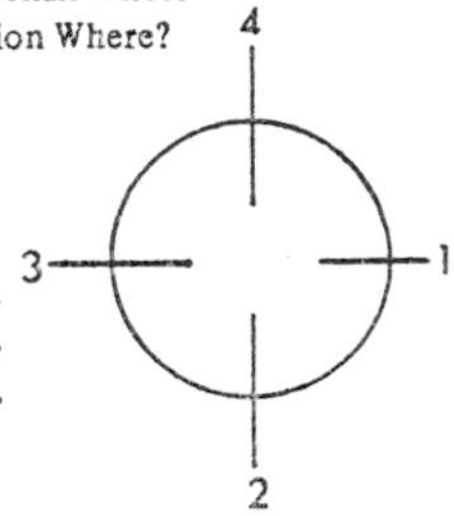

__(20)__   3. <u>Coordination:</u>
1. Walking and on all fours _____
2. Count coordinated with
movement_____
3. Sideways walk_____
4. Armswings (to waltz) _____

__(10)__   4. <u>Attention Span (Endurance):</u>
1. Hop and count _____ 2. Driving movement _____

__(10)__   5. <u>Physical Courage:</u>
1. Walk backward_____ 2. Roll back on floor
(Somersault)_____

__(35)__   6. <u>Ego Image:</u>
1. Lift on toes_____ 2. Stand on toes_____ 3. Walk on toes _____
4. Lift arms up _____ 5. Open arms out _____ 6. Lift head _____
7. Walk on toes, head up, arms _____

__(15)__   7. <u>Emotional State and Personality:</u>
Music stimulus_____Mental status_____Creative responses _____

__(130__   Total

Signed _____
Liljan Espenak, DTR

For additional notes use back page

Figure 3-7.

CHAPTER 4

TREATMENT, PHASE 1: RESTRUCTURING

PHYSICAL DYNAMICS

The TOTAL APPROACH of dance therapy is focused on the dynamics of body and mind in emotional interaction. There is a fundamental biological basis for this, as indicated by the basic cell reaction of the human body in terms of the relation between feeling and movement. Figure 4-1 illustrates this relationship.

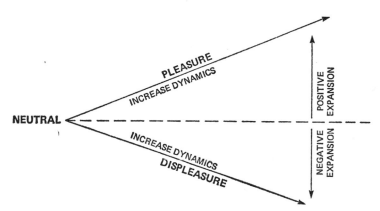

Figure 4-1. Basic cell reaction.

In feelings of pleasure, there is a basic cell reaction of expansion. In feelings of displeasure, the reaction is contraction. In awakening, for example, in a warm and pleasing room, there is a feeling of comfortable pleasure to which the basic cell structure responds with expansion; the same awakening in a cold, stiff, unattractive situation, with feelings of displeasure, would produce a body cell contraction. Thus, there is a continuous interplay on the biological level of the mental and the physical.

Because of these variances, this first phase of treatment consists primarily of physically therapeutic exercises, but the exercise itself is also designed to stimulate pleasurable use of body freedom to accelerate body cell expansion and, most importantly, to stimulate through specific exercise experience the awareness of the interaction between feeling and body expression.

We indicated in Chapter 1, that the treatment of this interaction of psyche and soma in dance can be traced back to the concepts of the classic Greek culture, and in Chapter 2 we brought this concept into its contemporary expression in both psychological theory and dance theory. There are, however, a number of equally historic concepts in regard to the use of special forms of exercise, as well as dance forms, that have been dedicated to the dynamics of personality and body integration. One of the major developments was in Dalcroze eurythmics, which considers psychological intervention an important part of their program in music education. Eurythmics emphasizes the benefits of rhythmic movement to music as a means of developing harmony between mind and body. Dalcroze eurythmics, which originated in Switzerland, is now part of the education curriculum in Swiss schools. Dalcroze was indeed one of the most relevant exponents of the interactive nature of physio/psychodynamism in exercise and gymnastic activities, and a brief review of his approach is valuable not only for a historical perspective but in understanding some of the technical aspects of dance therapy.

The fundamental principle of Dalcroze in music education is that theory should *follow* practice and that insight should *follow* experience. The practical objectives of his system of gymnastics is to develop the mind as a result of the physical experience and to achieve this by providing pupils with intense and continuous experience in movement to rhythm, to music, and to percussion. Dalcroze sought an immediate, continuing personal response to rhythms heard or felt. Similarly, in dance therapy we are not seeking to teach theory to our patients but rather to get that patient to experience his own body and to learn also about his mind and his feelings through this direct physical experience.

Dalcroze provided one of the highest forms of physical education in modern society and is one of the closest in approach to art form, comparable to dance itself. Dance therapy, in its evolutions from a base in psychology, takes this concept further through the therapeutic emphasis on the release of unconscious material and by its much stronger stress on personal spontaneity in movement.

In addition to the work of Dalcroze in this field, there are many other significant contributions, as discussed previously: the swing techniques of Bode and Medau in Germany; numerous American systems of exercise and relaxation; yoga techniques, with its emphasis on inner tranquillity. It obviously extends to the body-mind restructuring techniques in modern psychiatry, such as the work of Alexander Lowen in Bioenergetics and the theoretical formulations of Adlerian psychiatry.

Dance therapy itself is and should be eclectic—that is, it should draw upon the best and latest in physical education and dance as art form and from behavioral modification concepts in psychological and psychiatric theory. Dance therapy can also borrow effectively from certain concepts in oriental philosophy, such as Zen, which emphasizes the "letting go" of intellectual stress, an "emptying" of the mind, so that perceptive intuitions can rise from the deeper sources of awareness, and the body can then express these intuitions directly and spontaneously, as in Zen archery and fencing—both of which require the absolute unity of body and mind for expert performance.

The first phase, however, in the direction of mind and body unity or, to phrase it technically, toward body-ego harmony, is to get the patient to recognize his own body, and the exercise techniques are designed for this purpose, as well as for the correctional values. It is a method not only of restructuring posture and movement capabilities but of restoring self-confidence in the innate capacity of the individual to move expressively to his own inner rhythms, to respond freely to the stimulation of music and the movements of others, and to comprehend that the body is an expressive instrument used for the release of emotions.

Many individuals who are emotionally disturbed in relation to body image tend to have "dead" restricted areas within their body and its limbs, to show limited release of energy and drive, and to suffer from severe repression of emotions that they fear. Very frequently, there is an immediate reaction to the exercise techniques, such as heightened anxiety, weeping, or sporadic uncontrolled euphoria, as new body experience floods the personality that is not yet able to harmonize the stirring of habitual repressions. As true, deep feelings find their outlet through the body, these overt demonstrations alert the therapist to the individual's unconscious state and indicate the sources of the disturbance and the directions for therapy. As Freud once described the purpose of the dreams, we also see in expressive movement one of the detours by which repression can be avoided. Even in the first exercise phase, the experienced observer can detect the relationship among an individual's specific movements, his emotional response to those movements, and his affective state.

Strong emotional reactions to even simple postural adjustments can be expected. For example, in working a patient's shoulders to ease the stiff arms more naturally into the shoulder sockets, the transformation from closed, protected chest to exposed chest and open arms can bring about an outburst of anxiety. However, if the procedure is continued and habituated as physical experience, a sense of freedom will be developed, which itself produces a remission of the originally neurotic contractions and the blockage of the unconscious source.

Our emphasis now is addressed to the first phase of modification of body and movement behavior through a number of specific techniques, namely, to various forms of motor movement: balance, sacrum exercise, swings, and breathing.

EXERCISE TECHNIQUES

Forward Progression

The walk of an individual, constituting as it does the total involvement of body, limbs, posture, and movement, is the most important involuntary expression of that individual. The most critical area involved in the progression of the walk is the sacrum. The sacrum, the five fused bones at the end of the spine, is the center from which total body coordination, as expressed in walking, is initiated.

As the human infant develops from quadruped to biped, without any notable change in anatomical structure the complexity of retaining balance makes it more difficult to push the sacrum far enough back to allow it the freedom necessary for the smooth flow of movement downwards into the hind legs to propel them forward. Exercises to recapitulate this development of walk from quadruped to biped are one of the first treatments initiated for the patient, as it also is one of the first of the diagnostic tests. We introduce a series of arm and leg movements on all fours, in the opposition sequence shown in Figure 3-1.

We proceed with the continued practice of the motion in order to reach a smooth form in forward progression on all fours, where all steps interact and overlap harmoniously in a natural progression. As the quadruped step improves with practice, the body releases some of the energy in the "forelegs," or arms, to produce the rise to an upright position, just as man did in his original development from other mammals and apes.

With the body now in upright position, the forward walk is then practiced, maintaining the rhythm of oppositional arms and legs. When, with practice, the upright walk becomes smooth, the torso is then relaxed forward until hands touch the floor in the quadruped position. The quadruped walk is then repeated.

The total procedure is repeated from the quadruped walk to the biped walk and back again, all fours to upright to all fours, until the entire sequence can be performed evenly and harmoniously, without any interruption in the flow of movement. The upright walking movement is then followed for some time, to emphasize not only the practice but also the feeling of the even, smoothly progressing walk.

The role of the sacrum is, of course, essential to the development of harmony in motion. Photographs have been made of a sequence of walking steps, taken in darkness with a flashlight fastened to the hip of the walker. Figures 3-4 and 3-5 indicate this movement of the flashlight, and the consequent rolling movement of the pelvis in walking, demonstrating the circular motion of the free-swinging pelvis and sacrum. To develop this smooth circular movement, a number of exercises have been developed for the sacrum, which are performed lying down and they are outlined as follows:

Sacrum Exercise #1

(Sometimes referred to as "The Shrimp"; see Figure 3-2 A and B.)

Lie on side with arms overhead and legs outstretched.

1. Jackknife the body from the waist (the sacrum), leaving the legs and arms straight, and make hands and feet meet.
2. Straighten the body. Repeat. The movement must begin in the sacrum; the back and legs will follow. No force should be exerted from legs or from abdominal muscles.

Repeat movement. After completing the exercise once, turn over to other side and repeat.

Turn over to first side and repeat.

Sacrum Exercise #2

1. Repeat movement in exercise #1, but develop it to the degree where the forward movement ends in the fetal position.
2. Stretch extremities to the straight position, gradually arching the back, countermoving arms and legs to back. The important point to observe is the need for the upper and lower extremities to move in absolute coordination, whether the "jackknife" position is completely open, half closed, or completely closed.

Performing these exercises requires consciousness of muscular control, and this consciousness develops tension. The body must be allowed to submit to this conscious control and to tolerate the tension. With continued practice it then becomes possible to perform the movements by instinct without tension, and in a smooth and even manner.

Sacrum Exercise #3

Sacrum vibration in upright position. Vibration is a movement originating in the sacrum, which can vibrate the whole body if relaxation of the sacrum is achieved.

1. Stand with torso hanging forward, feet in second position, knees relaxed. Thighs hold weight of body over point of gravity; sacrum is highest point of back, yet it hangs loose.
2. Movement starts through sacrum pushing down to floor, making knees bend. In its returning movement, if relaxed, the circular motion of the pelvis reacts through the whole body. When repeated, the whole body becomes involved in a constant, slight vibratory movement. When achieved, the torso can slowly raise to upright. Furthermore, the weight can shift from one leg to the other. Once the weight shifting has been reached, the body can move forward or sideways or change the levels from high to low, maintaining the vibration throughout the body. Later goals are the fusion of these vibratory movements with a partner or in a group, producing a sensation of relaxed communion, as in the motions of primitive dance.

THE WALK. In all forms of forward progression the sacrum initiates the movement, as we have explored in the act of walking. When the sacrum moves downward, the foot is pushed along the floor; in the forward movement, the weight is transferred by the *back* foot. In the upward movement, the follow-through in the body by the thighs straightens it, and on the backward release, the released foot behind gets drawn in under the body in first position on its way through to the front again.

In the walk, the transfer of the weight is to the *whole* relaxed foot; for a brief moment during this movement, *both feet are on the floor* at the same time, which is distinctive to the act of walking.

THE RUN: As dynamics increase, the pushing motion of the feet become stronger. To counteract the push and cushion it, the knees and the ankles give way lightly, creating a slight bounce. In the run, only *one foot at a time is on the floor,* never both.

THE LEAP: With increasing dynamics, the running progression will no longer suffice. The energy of the sacrum has now become too great to retain the constant contact with the floor, and the body is catapulted upward by the rebounding energy of the foot. The step has now become a step in the air, *with both feet in the air* simultaneously, at some point in the sequence. The increase in dynamic drive, starting from the walking level, has taken the movement *upward* in space as well as forward. The result is a positive expansion toward two directions in space, which produces a sense of exhilaration and joy.

THE RUSH. Dynamic energy, however, may take a different direction into space—not only forward but *downward*. The drive, when increased in the downward direction, will change the walk into a fast-moving, rushing walk-run. To accomplish this, the knees must relax and allow the thighs to expand to their full length, increasing the size of the step.

THE TUMBLE: With further increase in drive downward, the rushing step, struggling with the dynamic demands and inhibited by the closeness to the floor, is forcefully changed to a *tumbling* forward motion. Figure 4-2 indicates the active dynamics.

There are also qualities that we consider passive in terms of locomotion dynamics, as illustrated by Figure 4-3. The passive quality of the movement changes the expression of the progression, which is achieved through placing the torso far back over the heels and leading with the pelvis. As before, the increase of energy drives the movements into the next spatial level, be that upward or downward, toward positive feelings or toward negative feelings; however, it has an entirely different—opposite— quality of expression from the active scale. These two scales of locomotion are significant indicators of the interaction among the elements of motivational drive in time and space through just the simplest of man's movements, i.e. forward progression.

Various types and variations in these progression possibilities are used for exploration of the patient's feelings and responses, i.e. backward progression, sideways movement, change of directions, interchange of movement levels, interchange of quality, active to passive.

While the therapist is observing and interpreting, the patient

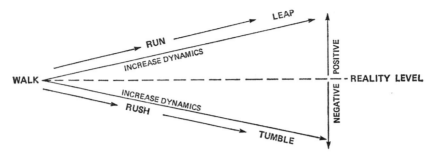

Figure 4-2.   Active scale of locomotion.

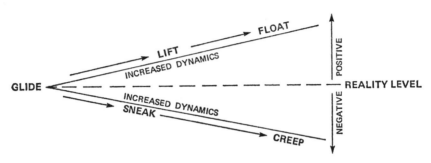

Figure 4-3.   Passive scale of locomotion.

is also observing and experiencing his own advances and retreats. He is beginning to understand that his body is expressing his feelings and his attitudes, his repressions and his releases, not always voluntarily. Moreover, throughout thcse fundamental experiences in progression on the reality level, and into explorations of space above and below the reality level, the patient is also involved, as is the therapist instructionally, in two additional aspects of progression and, indeed, all forms of movement, namely, posture and balance.

Posture

Man constantly copes with posture and balance in the universal relation of movement to gravity. When the body is stationary, there is, of course, natural positioning. If the stance is normal, from where the long arch in the foot meets the metatarsal arch to the crown of the head in standing position, the person is poised vertically in a 90° angle to the horizontal line of the ground. This stance is, in effect, determined by the same laws that govern all stationary bodies in relation to gravity. However, when movement occurs, the relationship shifts, as we all know, and certain conscious and unconscious adjustments are required to maintain placement and balance in relation to momentum and mass. While the ability to maintain balance through a varying complexity of movements and tempo is an innate capacity of the nervous system, lack of self-confidence, timorousness, and other emotional factors or attitudes interfere with an individual's capability to remain upright, as do defects in body control and in coordination. Therefore, attention must be given not only to the physical correctional techniques but also to the encouragement and other supportive activity of the therapist in freeing the individual from psychological obstructions to adjustment.

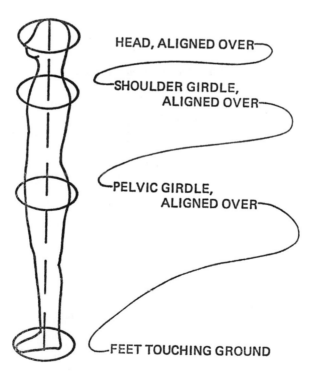

HEAD, ALIGNED OVER

SHOULDER GIRDLE, ALIGNED OVER

PELVIC GIRDLE, ALIGNED OVER

FEET TOUCHING GROUND

Figure 4-4. Posture placement.

Balance

The problem of balance first emerged when the human animal rose from quadruped to biped progression. Before progression could be attempted, balance had to be obtained in rising and standing. The gorillas and monkeys give us good demonstration of how that was accomplished in the evolutionary context. The human species, however, succeeded in remaining in the upright position as a result of environmental adaptation and related developmental factors; nevertheless, all individuals do not necessarily share the same degree of balance requisite for the smoothness of rising, standing, and moving functions.

The most obvious feature of the changes required for the transition in balance is the placement of the heaviest part of the body—the pelvis. The pelvis has to be counterbalanced by another heavy part—the head. It is clear that the pelvis, balanced over the feet, would require the head to be placed over the pelvis and the feet, which corresponds precisely with the laws of posture. In changing the walk from quadruped to biped and back again, this change of weight balance forward and back becomes very conscious, and the relationship of the pelvis, head, and shoulders as interrelated parts becomes a part of the physical realization.

With closed eyes, this recognition becomes stronger, and the inner certainty of the body parts' (pelvis, shoulder, head) relationship to gravity and erectness is learned, as in early childhood, through trial and error. With the new position, the feeling of the function of the feet in holding the body's weight and thus the contact with the earth becomes very apparent, and it constitutes an important condition for emotional security, parallel with the physical sense.

In developing this sense of security, one can consciously shift the weight and contact with the earth (floor, ground) from the front of the feet to the heels, from the outside of the feet to the inside, exploring the changes and the relief in returning to the secure placement over the long arch and metatarsal. From there, one can proceed to shifting from one foot to the other, from side to side, constantly reconfirming the contact with gravity, changing the shift from back to front and reversing.

The development of this is the constant shifting from the back foot to the front, i.e. walking. It then becomes obvious that the placement of the pelvis is the important condition for balance, as one feels the forward placement at each step. The thighs come strongly into play for this performance as they move over the metatarsal arches. (Refer to Figure 3-3 A, B, C, and D.)

There are many varied expressions of unbalanced walking, which are not always physically determined. A person in great haste will have the weight too far forward over the toes and almost fall over his feet (a head-over-heels example of imbalance). There are others who have developed a habit of overemphasizing the right side of the body, so they lead with their right shoulder and pelvis, giving them a sideways look. The very passive person will keep the weight so far to the back over the heels that the pelvis and abdomen are thrust forward to maintain balance. The person with a withdrawn (inhibited) pelvis must counteract this displacement by throwing shoulders and head back, thus creating the lordosis we so often see. All of these are faulty adaptations made for the unconscious purpose of adjusting an emotionally faulty balance.

Swings

By "swings" we mean all movements of the body that have a specific dynamic quality, where the swinging movement consists of an active impetus followed by a passive gradual depletion, in contrast to the vibratory movement that is maintained at a constant energy level. The momentum of the impetus in the swinging movement continues until all its force has been used, as in a pendulum swing. The movement sets up a wavelike action through the body creating an experience of harmony, of rhythmic awareness of vital energy.

Examples of swing movement exercises are the following:

1. Relax body, letting torso hang loosely, slightly forward over thighs and metatarsals, with knees slightly bent. Giving impetus at the hips and sacrum, push downward and forward in a semicircular line until the weight has shifted to the toes. Now release the down and forward thrust. The toes will take over the impetus and, fighting

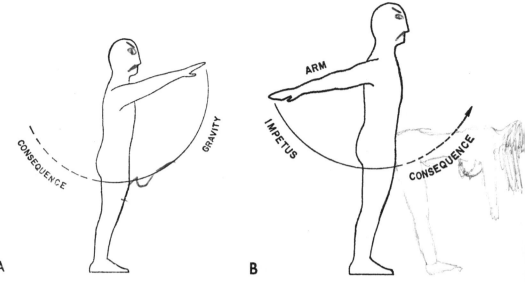

Figure 4-5.   Swing action. A. Gravity. B. Impetus.

gravity, will cause the pelvis to complete the missing upward and back semicircle. The rest of the body follows in wavelike motion; down and forward, up and backward.

2. Repeat movement, observing the action of the arms. The wavelike progression of movement through the torso carries into the arms, which in turn create their own circular movement.

3. Repeat movements a number of times until the coordination of the whole body creates a harmonious flow.

4. Repeat until the shifting of body weight becomes a natural and easy part of the organic process and until forward progression, while swinging, has been achieved.

5. Repeat the movement, adding more dynamic energy to the thrust of the sacrum. At the same time, let the arm-swing deliberately support the acceleration. The body will then progress in a skipping step through the impact of combined sacrum and arm swings.

The swing has a wide range of possibilities for combination. After the basic instinctual reaction to the pelvic thrust is accomplished, the arm action can create countless challenges through directional variations and also great emotional effect. At this point, however, we are discussing the movement as a major aspect of natural rhythmic dynamics, which offer an experience of integration between body and mind and which evoke a variety of somatic sensations, such as flowing, lifting, and sometimes a sense of cosmic unity.

It is through these experiences, which are predance experiences in natural locomotion without routine or rhythms, that the patient begins to experience his body through personal expression of movement in time and space. He begins to use his body to express his psychic charge in somatic idiom. He is releasing, although he may not yet know it, his inner stresses without the self-consciousness of verbalization.

Breathing

Control of breathing is the ability to regulate inhalation and exhalation of breath according to the pace at which movement is performed, as we see in the slow and deep breathing in relaxed movement and the quickened breath in rapid movements. Although the process of inhalation and exhalation that supplies the body with oxygen and removes waste and carbon dioxide occurs involuntarily, the ability to regulate the process consciously during the performance of a variety of physical movements at varying speeds and with varying degrees of dynamic drive is critically important to body efficiency in terms of maximum intake of oxygen to the bloodstream and brain with minimum strain.

In relaxation, control of breathing involves deep inhalations to insure flattening of the diaphragm muscle and maximum inspirations with gradual exhalations, thus making fullest use of the entire chest cavity in breathing. In active movement, such as sports, dance, and running, control of the breath requires short inhalations and exhalations throughout the performance. This conscious control is fundamental to stamina, coordination, and harmony in movement, as well as to the natural health processes of the body. The breathing rate in slow movement or in relaxation and the breathing rate in rapid movement may vary from

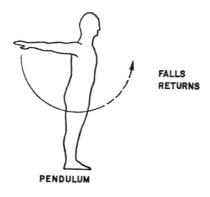

FALLS
RETURNS

PENDULUM

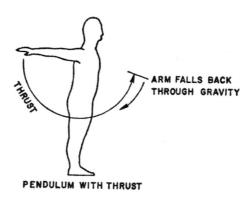

THRUST

ARM FALLS BACK
THROUGH GRAVITY

PENDULUM WITH THRUST

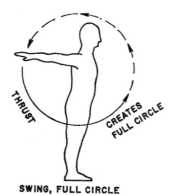

THRUST

CREATES
FULL CIRCLE

SWING, FULL CIRCLE

Figure 4-6.   Arm swing coordination; profile.

Dance Therapy

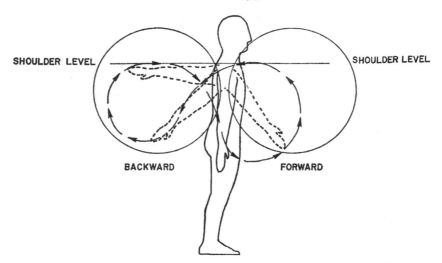

Figure 4-7. Swing, plain figure eight. Dotted lines represent the arm rotating from the shoulder in a circle forward and then backward, creating a form of the figure eight.

six to forty inhalations and exhalations per minute. The conscious ability to control and pace the breathing is a fundamental part of total body coordination in tension and in relaxation, and it is an essential part of the program for which we have specialized learning and correction techniques as part of the exercises.

It is through this restructuring program in motor movement, sacrum development, swings, placement and balance, and breathing that the patient begins to experience his body fully as a vehicle of movement in time and space. He is also beginning to use his body and its movements as release of emotional charge, and to the degree that he does this, the physical restructuring has begun to interact with unconscious processes. However, these events are often still occurring at the experience level, with less emphasis on the comprehension aspects of the therapy. While verbalizing thoughts and feelings does occur during interaction between therapist and patient, very often the major orientation during this restructuring phase is physical experience, with analysis following as changes occur in body image, self-concept, or feelings as an outcome of the direct physical approach.

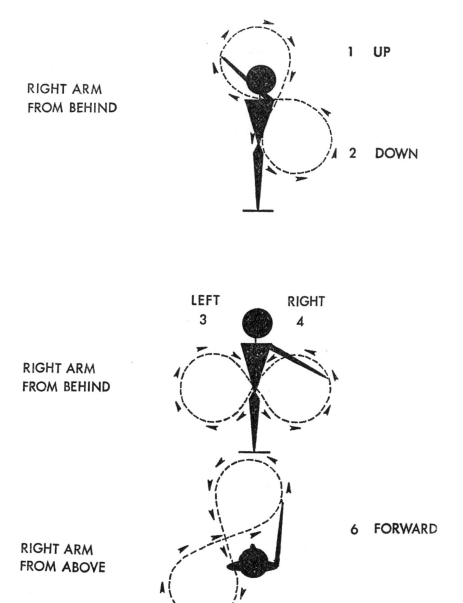

RIGHT ARM
FROM BEHIND

1 UP

2 DOWN

LEFT
3

RIGHT
4

RIGHT ARM
FROM BEHIND

6 FORWARD

RIGHT ARM
FROM ABOVE

5 BACKWARD

6 SWINGS IN SPATIAL DIRECTION

Figure 4-8. Spatial swings (according to Laban). Top: Vertical arm swing (up and down). Middle: Horizontal swings (in and out). Bottom: Arm swings in perspective (front to back). All of the swings are done in succession: up, down, in, out, back, front (1, 2, 3, 4, 5, 6).

It is, however, in the next phase of treatment (reviewed in the following chapter) that the work of integration between body and mind most clearly ensues. Emphasis is placed on total personality and improved harmony among emotional states, mental attitudes, and natural body movement.

CHAPTER 5

TREATMENT, PHASE 2: INTEGRATION

EMOTIONAL DYNAMICS

T HE RESTRUCTURING EFFORT, in the form of the early body work reviewed in the previous chapter, seeks primarily to improve coordination, stimulate realistic body awareness, and encourage body freedom. Our primary focus is to provide a structured opportunity of specialized exercises and rhythmic movements for the patient to experience his body in all its parts and as a unity and to become aware of such individual factors as strength, tension and relaxation, flexibility, balance, control, and all the related elements that constitute movement and that affect the natural harmony of neuromuscular inter-action. During this physically strengthening experience, which represents a departure from the patient's previously defensive behaviors and their accompanying physical restrictions, we have also opened up paths for emotional expression but have not yet sought specifically to elicit unconscious material.

Our basic psychological task in the exercises was to liberate the patient from anxiety and fear of his own motility, of his own physical dynamism. It is not motion itself of which he is afraid; he fears the emotions, associations, and the unconscious conflicts associated with movement in his self-concepts. He fears the power that freedom of movement represents, namely, the power to embrace or to destroy. Rather than experience these emotions and the punishing consequences that he thinks will follow, he has immobilized to varying degrees his vital energies and unconsciously selected parts of his body as threatening instruments of that energy. Within the structure and safety of the therapeutic setting, he can bring these fears and anxieties to the surface, where they can be consciously experienced and intellectually and emotionally assimilated and either resolved

79

or brought under control so that they no longer affect body image and body movement.

None of this is steady progress. There are various types of avoidance or denial behaviors, such as substitutions of movements, irrelevant movements and gestures, expressed or unexpressed reluctances to cooperate with the therapist in the physical areas, all of which are part of the struggle in self-confrontation and fear of change. We are more concerned with bringing the patient to the point where he overcomes his fear of movement and with preparing him for sensations of changes than in specifically eliciting the unconscious sources of his blocks. With the new experiences in both movement and the related satisfactions, certain modifications of the weak body image occur. We measure these changes at intervals by readministering the diagnostic tests and charting the comparison between initial performance and successive movement behavior as the treatment process continues. Moreover, a relationship between therapist and patient is developed. We are observing the degree of resistance and the forms that this resistance takes; we are acquiring a more profound grasp of the unconscious dynamics powering that resistance and have developed an overall effective working sensitivity to the needs and problems of the patient.

The next phase of treatment, which we are concerned with in this chapter, is devoted to the task of integrating the unconscious fears, repressed emotions, and associations into consciousness and restoring the patient as fully as possible to a unified body-ego state. The major technique used for these objectives in dance therapy is to stimulate authentic feelings through individual dance or improvisations, insofar as they have not already appeared as associations during the first phase of the program. The role of improvisation in dance therapy is of the utmost significance to effective treatment and is reviewed in detail in the following discussion.

IMPROVISATION

Free improvisation is a most vital element in treatment because of its inherent power to draw out the patient's emotional content with or without conscious volition. It has the function of embodying the feelings and of bringing them to the surface, where their force can be experienced as the dynamic underlying body-ego disturbance.

This improvisation as a therapeutic technique is not always simply a matter of the patient's dancing in any form at will. It is important to understand that the therapist is professionally in control of the stimulation offered. Improvisation in the technical sense is free movement in response to specifically selected stimuli, which are based on professional appraisal of the problems and needs of the patient. For example, in selecting certain types of music or percussion rhythms as stimulus for dance improvisation, the therapist would select different types of sound pattern and tempo for a hyperactive, overstimulated patient in whom the ability to control movement or to sustain stillness or repose was sought than he would select for an overly passive patient from whom an active kinetic response was sought. For a depressed patient, we would want to be able to offer stimulation of feelings of joy or freedom that would penetrate the depressive armor, and so on. These examples are, of course, oversimplifications of the problem and the task, but they serve to demonstrate the point that each case will require its own forms of stimulation for dance improvisation, which are based on the sensitivity and experience of the therapist. This sensitivity to the individual psychological constellation must accompany the total treatment process but is particularly critical in the choice of improvisational techniques where we are dealing with the release of unconscious feelings as a function of personality integration.

The major categories of stimulation that we employ in improvisation treatment are the following:

1. Music—Melody
2. Music—Rhythm (Drums and Other Percussion Instruments)
3. Symbolism and Free Fantasy
4. Images and Emotional Dynamics of Everyday Life

Music—Melody

Virtually every form of music can be used for stimulation of dance improvisation or movement employing both spontaneous and directive approaches. The sound of music has a number of therapeutic applications: it may overcome self-consciousness in regard to dance movement or inhibition in the presence of others; it may serve as a catalyst in activating unconscious memories and associations; it may stimulate new moods and impulses; it can revive or intensify emotional states; and most importantly, it can provide a pleasurable sensory and kinetic experience.

Music is inherently persuasive. It does not require sophistical cultural awareness to produce its "magic" effects. Sound itself evokes memory and association, going back to sounds heard very early in life: the lullaby, the footsteps outside the nursery door, the birds outside the window, the bark of the family dog. All of these negative and positive sound experiences have become part of the unconscious auditory memory, along with the sounds of nature, the roar of the sea, the peal of thunder, the rush of the tree branches in the wind. Even in sophisticated forms, music may arouse elemental memories, induce revery, and awaken emotions long repressed. Our hearing does serve as a form of emotional as well as intellectual communication, and it is common experience that certain sounds produce universal and individual response. A foghorn at night sounds eerie and sad. There is a contagion of mood between the sound and the hearer, and reverberations of common feelings are produced within us with the sound of a brass band (aggression), the sound of rain (calmness), snowfall (peace), the sound of crying (pity, compassion).

In considering its therapeutic application, we are concerned not only with the direct response but with the associations that accompany that direct response. Human emotions do not constitute simple, discrete, direct experiences; rather, they consist of a network of experiences, which are highly individualistic, in which the primary feeling is linked with many related subordinate feelings that are all attributes of the emotion most closely perceived. Similarly, music in its organization can be equally complex. Silences, increases and diminutions of sound, accelerating or slowing of tempo, and all the other components of the organization of music strike their corresponding vibrations in the listener, producing an interaction of music-emotional experience that constitutes a very critical technique in the therapy. Music is a technique used to stimulate catharsis in the patient, hopefully surfacing in movement, where it can become sufficiently conscious to effect behavior changes.

Music—Rhythm

The concept of rhythm is distinct from that of music in the context of therapeutic considerations, since rhythm is most potent in its direct, noncerebral stimulation of instinctive body response. We seek to reach the personal rhythms inherent in individuals through a wide range of rhythmic sounds from the primitive to the sophisticated. For this purpose, we utilize a variety of percussion instruments and rhythm patterns, incorporating the techniques of many cultures, borrowing from the East as well as from our own contemporary rock culture. Rhythm is the special province of percussion instrumentation, evoking spontaneous physical response as well as the complex introspective experience. The simplicity of form and the repetitive quality of the motifs make it particularly persuasive to the listener and provide a simple way for him to absorb the sound and make it part of himself. The patient can "give in" to rhythm yet retain form and control in his responsive movement.

In working with the patient, we become increasingly aware of his sensitivities to different types of mood-inducing rhythms. Slow rhythms can be reflected in responses of sadness, hesitancy, and calmness. Fast rhythms can be exhilarating or can create anxiety or even fear. Between these extremes there are varying degrees of positive or negative reactions that release the dynamic energy of the patient. Primitive drum beats may encourage the expression in movement of assertive, aggressive, or even hostile uses of energy; strong hard beats on the gong can bring feelings of grandiosity or power to the surface or can produce the full motion of swinging or whirling in joyous or trancelike abandon. Small drums can be used to stimulate excitement, tension, exuberance, or, at the other end of the spectrum, an apprehensive rigidity. Monotonies, created by the use of gongs, cymbals, wooden drums, and other percussion instruments can create a certain hypnotic monotony, and they are also a means of gliding from activity into passivity. The sound concentration, the simplicity of its emotional color, and the prolonged repetition calm the body down. Without it being perceived, the feeling of balance increases through the repetitive movement, and fears are diminished. When circular swings of the torso are performed as a group in a sitting position, the reinforcement derived from the movement of others combined with the monotony of the rhythm becomes so intensified that some of the participants slide out on the floor in relaxed sleep. This overall relationship among rhythms, instruments and emotions is, in fact, a significant field of study in itself for the dance therapist.

There is another area where the dynamics of rhythm are powerfully employed, i.e. *personal rhythms*, which effect the discovery of self and the improvement of self-image. The inner rhythms of an individual are characteristic of the personality; this individual rhythm is not generally known even to the emotionally healthy individual, although it is observable in the affirmative harmony and balance of his appearance and movements. In the disturbed person, the developmental deficits in ego formation are accompanied by elements of disintegration in the basic life rhythm. During the therapy process, we try to restore to the patient a sense of his natural rhythm—a sense that he will acquire not only from his adaptations to external rhythms but also from our observation of his breathing during improvisation. Training in breathing is part of the treatment process so that the patient learns to develop a harmony between energy expenditure and breathing behavior. Dance improvisation to rhythm, which accentuates the rhythm of the breathing patterns not only in movement but in the emotional reactions as well, is important in the learning of proper breathing in relation to the tension and relaxation of movements and feelings. We seek to make contact with the patient's internal rhythms by coordinating with his pulse beat and by observing his breathing at the emotional and the physical level; in anger, the rhythm will be short and percussive; in fear, suppressed; in joy, accelerated but regular, in calm, slow and deep. If the patterns are inappropriate and if restricted breathing is due to emotion-inhibiting practice, the focus on breathing and its relationship to individual personality rhythm may open up areas for further exploration of the unconscious for the work of integration.

Symbolism and Free Fantasy

The foregoing chapters explained that personality has not developed in a vacuum and that both conscious thinking and feeling are the building factors. One of the still untapped sources of emotional response becomes available to us through symbolism, religious and philosophical influences, and free fantasy.

We express our moods by our facial expression and our attitudes and feelings by movement and gestures so precise that others recognize them more accurately from our body dynamics than from our words. The same facility of interpretation applies in the case of the universal symbol as it does to individual symbolization, since we find the same connection between mental and physical experience. The universal symbol is ever-present in dance. A few of the well-known symbolic gestures are folded hands in prayer, touching the forehead in blessing, hand on heart for love, tap of forehead for "crazy," cross the heart for honesty.

For creative improvisations, however, the symbolic meaning is more hidden, and thus more subtly answered. The "dancers" search unconsciously for the definition of the underlying mood, explore the phases of their own self-discovery as they delve down into the wellspring of feeling. Intuitively, they will raise a finger and point to heaven. They may rock a baby; they may stretch out both arms, forming a cross with their body. They may crouch in grotesque expression of some untold hell; they may show purity in the lines of the lotus flower.

Through the reciprocity of mind and body these intuitive movements can all be used as central themes in body representation. Improvisations serve a purpose in treatment by revealing the significant symbolic message. Conversely, these physical phenomena can suggest emotional experience through the age-old symbols of humanity, presented as a form of direct stimulation to activate patient response, for example, such symbols as fire, water, air, crown of kingships, tower of isolation, snake, light, black clouds, and rainbow. There are plant symbols, animal symbols, and color and number symbols, each in their indicated place. Fairy tales may come to the fore and be relived in a new light of personal meaning. Obscure myths arise and become understood as the realities of time and space are dispersed, and the "dancer" draws upon ancient lore, wisdom, and associations to express his personal truths in response to universal symbols.

Images and Emotional Dynamics of Everyday Life

To use an image as stimulus for movement or movement references is to approach emotions via the intellect, while music, rhythm, and symbols appeal directly to the emotional life. Verbal communication—that is, the presentation of selected images for responsive improvisation—is addressed, although not exclusively, to our perception and intellectual understanding. It does not end on that level, however. One also reacts with feelings.

In cases where exposure to the incomprehensible impact of music might be rejected, the road of logic remains open. Words, for many, stand for concrete things, for reality itself, for what you can pragmatically see and know as truth. While words in this sense are factual, they can also describe images and evolve fantasies. Words can come alive as they venture into the realms of the imagination. If one more step is taken, we arrive at identification, which is always associated with feelings. For example, the therapist might present a very broad and universal image such as "the sea" or some of the other word pictures discussed. Obviously, the immediately recognizable permits an enormous range of individual expression in movement. The universality of the image "the sea" might evoke first perhaps a series of conventional wavelike or swimming movements but would then develop in dance beyond the purely imitative or representative aspects into movement expression of images reflective of individual feelings, memories, and associations. How many different images and emotions could be expressed in reference to the image of the sea? (1) The experience of a beautiful day at the beach; (2) a stormy and threatening experience; (3) a feeling of wonder and awe at the vast expansion to distant shores; (4) danger of shipwreck and apprehension of death; (5) the search for sunken treasures; (6) the teeming life of the depths; (7) scuba diving and exploration of sea caves; (8) the charms of the dolphin or the danger of the shark; (9) gathering shells on the beaches; (10) sailing, cruising, all sorts of boating experiences. These ten obvious examples of personal image associations can be stimulated by one word, sea. In response, feelings emerge of peace, fury, majesty, fear, curiosity, excitement, playfulness, charm, gentleness, and power. Each individual adds his personal stamp to the improvisation as he experiences himself moving from the purely representational interpretation to the personal evocation of his private image.

The improvisation becomes, from the very nature of inner associations, not simply an interpretation of the patient's idea of the sea but an exploration of the self as the patient yields to the imaginative power of this concept. The dynamics involved are similar to the experience of reading poetry, where at a certain point, the feelings and projections of the reader are stirred beyond the ordinary comprehension of the words. It is the world of the indefinite within the definite that leaves the road open for the expression of authentic individual feelings.

For a more complex approach in relation to the personality needs and intellectual sophistication of the patient, we may draw upon poetry, legend, and mythlogy to provide an imaginative dance situation upon which the patient can express his images in free association, the starting of a train of thought, and movement, which then carries the "dancer" into his own personal realm.

Basically, the use of all or any of these images serves to move the patient from the voluntary level of association to the involuntary level as he stirs more closely to the fantasies and phantoms of his inner life. To recall and reexperience the sensations of stored impressions with the body as physical instrument is to reexperience onself in the present. The intellect only chooses the main theme; the memory and the unconscious become involved, each memory carrying with it a river of other memories, hopes, and possibilities that were previously unrecognized and unexplored. The specific image chosen, either by the therapist or by the patient, is simply a catalyst to evoke psychological interaction focussed on the therapeutic goal.

In the context of the dynamics of everyday life, we may introduce more realistic and concrete forms of stimulation, as the body-ego balance becomes more equalized in the course of treatment. We would employ the ordinary conflicts of life itself, for example, those which relate to direct physical experience. Introducing *definite actions,* such as "rebellion," "flight," "fight to win," "ice that melts," "push your way through the crowd," "walk against the wind," or other motivational actions rather than image orientations, indicate the patient's mode of coping with stress situations in life. Moreover, subjects such as these allow a follow-through of a conflictual situation, since its resolution can be seen in dance.

In using this technique, it is necessary that the therapist select situations of direct relevance to the patient's problems, level of intelligence, and milieu. The improvisational topics may range from conflicts in relationships and circumstances to personal aspirations and emotional behaviors, such as passivity or aggression. The main point is to select an interaction that is personally relevant to the patient. Wisely employed, the technique is effective in stimulating the flow of psychodynamics, which involve the personality at all levels—mind, body, emotions, and behavior on the plane of reality.

INTEGRATION

As the foregoing discussion of four major techniques used in dance improvisation indicates, we view the total improvisation technique as a methodology for eliciting the *involuntary* release of emotions and memories. It is a technique for evocation. Even if the patient is consciously denying or concealing feelings, the body will speak for itself in the progressive response of movement. As hitherto repressed or denied feelings come to the surface, the patient develops a more profound awareness of the self. *Unless he reaches himself at the psychic level, there can be no complete change,* only certain improvements that he is deriving from the physical restructuring process.

This approach, of course, is not different in principle from those in the verbal forms of therapy, where the analysis of dream content, free association, and so on, is used to surface unconscious material with the objective of ultimate integration with the total personality. Dance therapy, however, provides through improvisation a direct access to a body expression that transcends the conscious personality mechanisms of the patient. The use of such influences as music, rhythm, and imagery provides a *sensory* persuasion of mind and body to respond. It could be said that the powers inherent in the spell of music, rhythm, symbol, and fantasy are *seductive* toward unconscious elements in the personality, that they are evocative at the sensory level in a manner that cannot be matched by the powers of the intellect alone. It is at this sensory level that we capture the body response, which in turn brings mind and psyche with it, since there cannot be any separation among these elements. Dance itself, even in its most rudimentary forms, is an expression of personal feeling, using as its instrument the body, creating its patterns in space and time. In therapy dance encompasses not only the action of the mover but also the subjective concept of the mover plus the interpretation of the observer. When the patient experiences his body moving differently than before, his ideas about that body also change. When he is in visual positions that he has never experienced before, he sees the setting around him, the physical environment, also changing within the new angles of his vision. When he makes different kinds of thrusts and directions into space, he perceives new dimensions in space. When he moves in differing tempi to differing rhythms, he feels a new sense of time within his body and his mind.

Dance is not simply a question of discharging energy in impulses of fantasy or feeling, it is a total impact upon perceptions. Consequently, unless his fear of new perceptions immobilizes him completely, as in severe neurotic and psychotic states or his intelligence is so impaired that he cannot integrate these new perceptions with his consciousness, as in retardation, these new perceptions of body, movement, time and space will progressively expand the previous limitations of the body-ego concept.

Let us take for an example one of the improvisation techniques previously reviewed—the use of rhythm by percussion instruments: (1) The sounds of rhythm produce a response tension in the body. The response results in the creation of a form of movement in time and space. (2) The sudden sound of the gong or the clash of cymbals interrupts the rhythm, enveloping the dancer in space quivering with sound (3) The rhythm on the drums begins again, in crescendo, stimulating increased tensions and activating greater energy of movement. (4) Then, retardando, and the speed and action decreases, fading away into silence, emptied of activity. Out of these alternating sensory and motor experiences there is a transmission of energy that creates specific discharge of body and mind response. The moods and associations that accompany this movement transform passivity into action; thus, the body impulse and the emotional energy are both discharged in an experience of body-mind unity, a felt harmony between the action of the body and the impulse of the ego. As these connecting experiences continue, supported by the therapist, the process of integration of unconscious elements into consciousness occurs, with corresponding modifications of personality.

CHAPTER 6

EXPRESSIVE MOVEMENT IN GROUP INTERACTION

GENERAL CONSIDERATIONS

T HE PROCESS OF self-integration while it represents the major phase of treatment, is not the total objective of the therapy. It is, rather, the constructive process by which the patient is strengthened to achieve the ultimate goal, i.e. to live more comfortably and productively in the world of functions, tasks, aspirations, and relationships.

As the final phase of the treatment, the patient may join the group therapy program. This group dance setting offers an effective opportunity for both continued self-expression and modification of that self-expression in appropriate consideration and adaptation to the needs of others. Communal dance forms, as discussed earlier, are one of the historical expressions of group *identity* and group *communication.* One of the simplest approaches is to unite the group, as indicated on the discussion of primitive folk dance in Chapter 1, through response to rhythms. Within this setting, leadership may evolve from within the group itself, thus permitting various personalities to develop their own roles within the group. In the context of leader/follower formations, each personality will reveal himself at once; the aggressive personality will seek dominance, the competitive personalities will challenge; the passive personalities will follow; the isolated personalities will tend to withdraw or avoid.

The group then becomes a model world, reproducing on its own scale the interactions of personality in the world outside. Being able to function as member or as leader, or alternately fulfilling the respective demands of either role in this model world, will strengthen identity concepts, which in turn will

modify behavior in the real world. The patient learns to accept
or tolerate the attitudes and roles of differing personalities. He
develops increased awareness of the rights and boundaries of
others, as well as of his own, and most importantly, he learns
how to contain or to release his feelings in socially acceptable
ways. The pressures of a peer group, both affirmative and negative, supply effective motivation for the modification of social
behavior.

Technically, the dynamics in a mixed group might take form
along these lines, although it must be stressed that every session
differs and the following is only one example: The leader offers
the group the choice of music. If the group is unresponsive,
the leader tries to be sensitive to the mood of the majority and
makes the music selection accordingly. Sometimes if the mood
is depressed, the choice of music may mirror that mood, as a
starting point, from which point the dynamics of the session
would move upwards. But more frequently, the group would
suggest popular music—rock, jazz, waltz, polka, acording to group
population.

The leader opens his arms and offers his hands to the groups
in an invitation to form a circle or parallel formations on each
side. In either of these formations, the group initially performs
simple, rhythmic movements, not yet attempting partnerships;
the objective is to achieve first a strong group formation. In
counteraction, one or more members may break out of the
formation, either to withdraw or to start an individual set of
movements to the music. It then becomes a matter of the leader's
sensitivity to try to restore individual dancers to the formation or
to move the group around the new leader. The option of any
member to become a new leader is always open, as new formations occur. As the session proceeds, the pace of the activity is
quickened; the group may dissolve into individual improvisations
or couple dances and then reunite at the end of the session in
circle dance.

The great variety of new movement patterns, with music or
without, awakens and constantly renews the interest in the
activity of motion in space through encounters, parallel movements, circle formations, group vibrations, progression on the

three different levels (high, middle, and low), increase and decrease in speed, as will all the imagery made available by the leader. The group may concern itself with expressing in movement a dynamic subject, such as "turning their backs on each other and then facing," "sticking one's head out," "trip the light fantastic together," "cohesion," or "leadership and dependency." By experimenting with evolving a leadership from within a group, for example, each individual's reaction to this problem comes immediately to the fore as described earlier. In the "trip the light fantastic together," a two some or three-some, or the whole group, may have a hilarious time together, romping around the room and letting inhibitions go. There will be resistance from some even in this, as always, convincingly demonstrated in visible movement, and thus giving an opening for free discussion of the problem by the whole group.

There is, of course, a focus in group dance therapy on accommodation and communication. These goals, professionally supported by the therapist, make it possible to develop interactional contact among those who for a variety of reasons have difficulties in social contact. In order to communicate in this setting, the patient must develop an awareness of his own body signals as well as the desire and ability to understand the postural and movement communications of others. He must also develop his desire and capacity for coordinating his movements with that of others and adapting his inner rhythms to that of others. The focus, therefore, is greatly on accommodation, which in turn is undertaken to develop social expansion and competence. The capacity for moving in coordination with others is a fundamental one for person-to-person interaction, whether it be walking down the "street" in parallel movement or moving in a circle with a group. This coordination is necessary to the beginning of an encounter with another, the maintenance of the encounter and the disengagement of the encounter. Developing readiness and ease in these transactions is therefore one of the goals of the group therapy experience.

The material to draw from is inexhaustible; interaction, communication, withdrawal, frustration, sharing, tolerance, acceptance of criticism and, indeed, the total interplay of group dynamics that we recognize in the psychotherapeutic situation are here expressed in movement and movement sensitivity.

Within the framework of large muscle movement, there are a number of more subtle skills: recognition of the basic readiness between two people to encounter, necessity for vis-à-vis facial and eye contact, adjustment of the bodies in space, time, and direction, ease in touching and holding. All of this occurs, whether in group or couple dance, since in all these conditions there is always the "other." Moreover, choices are being made of whom to stand next to in the circle, whom to choose or accept in the couple dance, and whom to dance for, often unconsciously, in the improvisation.

It is obvious that if an individual is persistently unaccommodating he will be less and less desirable as companion in group or partner in couple dance. These "rejections" lead to frustrations that the patient has to work out in the group dance situation. Patterns of behavior then appear, which become a focus for the therapist, with a view in restoring to the patient his capacity for interaction. It is equally obvious that if his availability can be developed through treatment for adjusting to sharing time, space, and direction with others he will be developing an attitude and skill of vital importance to his life as a socialized human being.

In restructuring and improvisation the emphasis on individual therapy is on release of aggressions, fears, and constraints; in group therapy the emphasis is on not denying or repressing these feelings but on controlling them in the social situation *along with conscious recognition of the inner feelings.* In short, the experience in the group dance sessions can be considered social behavior therapy with the body as instrument—a necessary supplement to the task of inner integration, which is not complete until a corresponding translation of that inner harmony can be offered to others.

Dance therapy group sessions also employ the many techniques currently offered in the sensitivity workshops and weekend encounter marathons. In fact, these movements have originally been inspired by modern dance education, which uses them as part of their body awareness and training for working in dance companies, and they were common practice before the sensitivity workshops appeared on the psychology scene. Obviously, in order to maintain your placement on a stage during performances, it is essential to be fully aware of everyone else around you and their placement, tension, and interactive relationship to you. These are qualities much needed for function in the world as well. Thus, they are part of our therapeutic techniques.

We also use more sophisticated psychomotor techniques, as developed in ongoing dance therapy groups of neurotic patients. Intellectual and emotional demands may be greater in such a group, and insight may be more rapidly obtained. The group members are viewers as well as role players in the therapeutic constellation, which allows a fuller participation and meets many deeper needs of the patients.

For example, the problem of attachment is clearly visualized when two people are literally tied to each end of a rope and thus are being inhibited in movement and dynamics. The character of each individual will become evident, i.e. the dominant party will take over, or there may be a tussle, or both may roll in towards each other, mutually seeking contact and support. Sometimes the rope is closed and two or three participants are inside the circle of the rope. There will be differences in the balance of the three, two to one, or even each as equal entities. The restriction of the rope can become unbearable to one and can make that individual aggressively attack the other two, two might join in suppressing the third, or two might join in helping the third party if he is weaker. This type of discovery of one's individual actions to stress on the physical plane can be used as a basis for psychological change.

As another example, starting from separate corners, two or three participants can move in free improvisation, allowing for intuitive approach in movement to one or the other. Personal empathy and manner of approach is disclosed; jealousy may be exhibited, along with rejection and competition. These feelings are then dealt with in the discussion following. Often all three patients may be able to find a threesome unity.

A further example may occur when one of the participants

has realized a character problem that he has struggled to over-come. A case in question was the habit of evasion. Whenever confronted with difficulties, this patient would always evade the issue, either by leaving the scene or outwardly agreeing with the opponent. It became clear that she was suffering from a deep-seated fear of losing the battle, of being criticized, rejected, or penalized. All this was displayed on the physical plane in her preference to yield rather than fight. A movement situation was devised in which the group would function as the opponent, challenging this patient at her every move, pursuing her to the corner of the room, and not allowing her to escape. Under such pressure and without a way of retreat, she finally mobilized all her aggression and faced the group squarely, possibly for the first time in her life recognizing, feeling, and using her inherent strength.

Other techniques encompass improvisational work with eyes closed, fostering great sensitivity in touching. It is possible to have five people moving with closed eyes, and intuitively find each other, creating a "pyramid of unity" without ever opening their eyes. The technique of vibration done together can bring a group of even ten to twelve patients into a cohesive unit. Any deviation in rhythm in the group, no matter at which place in the line or circle, is felt by the others, and a "tuning in" must follow to unify the rhythms of the entire group.

It is clear from this discussion that the therapist must not only be aware of a wide variety of techniques but also have the sensitivity to the appropriateness of their application, both in cases of great sophistication as well as on the simplest intellectual level or, in the case of language problems, as the following story may illustrate.

I was travelling in Japan and scheduled to speak at a school for the mentally retarded in Kobe on the invitation of Kobe City Hall. During a tour of the school's facilities, we were shown into a classroom where the teacher was playing some simple folk tune on the piano. The class was listening without any sign of participation.

On the suggestion of the superintendent, I moved toward a child in the middle of the group and moved my hands in a figure eight, from the wrist, in rhythm with the music. The child followed my movement with his eyes, and when I opened my hands in front of him, he put his hands in mine. Together we moved our hands to the music, up and down, apart and together, and ended with the music, laying the hands to rest on the table. Instantly the child next to him held out his hands for me to "dance" with him, and each child then in turn held out his hands for his turn, until I had moved with each one of the twelve children present. Only one out of twelve did not respond.

I do not speak Japanese nor did the children speak English, yet there was complete human understanding, a perfect basis for therapeutic relationship.

SPECIALIZED GROUP APPLICATIONS

The previous review of some of the techniques used in group dance therapy apply, on the whole, to relatively "normal" patients who have different syndromes of body-ego imbalance but who are normally intelligent, are free from various forms of either mental or physical pathology, and can respond in varying degrees to the types of group stimulation offered. There are, however, a number of situations where the group approach must be radically modified; for example, different approaches must be used in dance therapy groups of mentally retarded patients, patients with sensory impairment in vision or speech, brain-damaged patients, the severely emotionally disturbed, and such special age groups as the geriatric or the very young.

To illustrate these specialized group applications, we will review two of the more experimental settings: (1) group therapy with psychotic ward patients, (2) group therapy with elderly patients in the nursing home setting. Obviously, both of these very different situations require adaptive or innovative approaches.

Stress Reduction with High Risk Ward Management Problems

Work with high risk patients has been undertaken at the Stress Reduction Learning Center at Creedmore, which was founded in 1974 by Mark Stebbins. The approach is based on the original work by Dr. Seymour Halpern and supplemented to include psychomotor skills, perceptions, and socializations. Dance therapy, therefore, has become an important contribution to the program.

"High risk ward problems" may be defined primarily as hyper-activity, autism, self-abuse, schizophrenia, paranoia, and aggressive behaviors. The utility of dance therapy in this framework relates to a stress reduction concept that views the problem of unconscious repression as inseparable from neuromuscular contingents and that the psychic conflicts can be approached by postural means. This specifically somatic approach corresponds with both psychomotor therapy and with bioenergetics.

The relaxation technique of shoulders and head, which was described earlier, is here applied in an extended form. An individual who is unable to organize his thoughts to process information about his physical environment is generally unable to articulate his physical movements. Relaxation techniques are one of the means of helping such patients focus upon attention to the environment and to others and giving them a basis for perception. Consequently, the emphasis in this experimental program is to use relaxation techniques by placing patients in a supine position and guiding them, through applied breathing techniques, to become absolutely still. Thus, the first part of the physical program was to achieve relaxation, for whatever period it could be sustained, and to create a controlled but casual and permissive atmosphere, where patients were free to leave or to reenter the group situation during any of the sessions.

Faced with such a challenging population (eight severely disturbed patients), the first effort had to be directed exclusively toward establishing a positive relationship with the members and motivating them to participate.

One of the patients, A (syndrome: blind obedience and echolalia), through the willingness to follow, created a model of what "dance" therapy might be and enabled the others to watch. Only two (A and B) of the eight patients present joined the movements, but with them it was possible to swing the arms, bend and stretch the torso, do knee bends, head movements, big and small steps. Together they did the pushing-pulling rocking-boat movement (which requires cooperation), after which their interest waned. Another patient, C (autistic), then spontaneously joined the others on the floor without doing any exercises, but he sat there for a short period until, suddenly and swiftly, he left the room. One of the girls, D, watched from another room and went in and out of the dance room a few times. When invited to join, she ran away. Another girl, E, rejected any contact initiated but responded with "goodbye" when the session ended. In spite of the difficulties, some contact with these highly isolated individuals was being made.

During the following weeks, the pattern of the sessions was much as indicated, with gradual spontaneous but sporadic participation by one or the other of the patients. One patient, F, wandered around, grabbed the hands of the therapist, moved them up and down, coming closer and closer, before darting from the room; another, G, came to observe for two or three times before he decided to participate. When he finally did, he sustained his participation in the movements for almost an hour.

Gradually, with the improvement in attention, new movements were introduced, and "grounding" was attempted. The important function of bending knees for elasticity and the full experience of pushing or kicking the floor away were introduced, giving the patients an unconscious feeling and experience of gravity (one of our original sources of security), and stretches toward the ceiling were done, reaching out and slowly sinking to the floor (the floor becomes a friend that can receive us for resting). The structure of the sessions had to change constantly from complete freedom of choice to voluntary control in organized movement consciously selected for the individual's problem. For work in a group situation in the wards, the individual approach takes place in the form of emphasis on certain techniques needed by individual members. It almost becomes several individual sessions within a group. The advantage here is that the group is available for socializing by working in twos and threes, for a more communal feeling, when possible, or for supplying a group experience even for those who were not specifically participating in a given session.

At the end of seven months' weekly sessions, three of the

patients had become available for a directed program, namely, patients A (echolalia), D (schizophrenia), and G (paranoia), because all three had shown noted improvement.

Patient A had made the greatest physical strides, advancing in awareness and animation, initiating ideas on his own, becoming quite lively, and smiling often.

Patient D had originally wandered in and out of the room, but by the fifth session she decided to stay and participate. First, she was walking around in a circle talking to herself of her fears, hates, and violent urges, but finally she calmed down enough to go through a series of arm movements, which signified the beginning of her participation. In the following sessions, although she was continually agitated, she continued to make the effort, learning to relax on the floor and asking the therapist to write down the exercises for her. Ultimately, she began to show signs of real pleasure in attaining skill and building confidence with this new emotional experience.

Patient G, who was extremely hyperactive, was treated with the calming techniques of rhythms and ultimately made verbal contact with other members, becoming more receptive to movement instruction. During the last session, G showed more recognition and awareness and had become much more mobile with his arms. When he again lay down on his mat, a new exercise was tried, interchanging tension and relaxation in a contracting and stretching sequence done on the side. (Refer to Figure 3-2 A and B.) This relaxed him so completely that he remained on the floor, very still, without his hair-twining motion, for a full ten minutes. This was impossible to expect at the beginning of the treatment.

Naturally, with such seriously disturbed patients, these incremental changes are a promise of continued improvements in dance therapy. The program is experimental, but it indicates one of the very specialized applications of psychomotor approach to intervention with otherwise inaccessible patients.

Dance and Psychomotor Therapy for a Geriatric Population

Dance therapy offers a considerable potential for meeting some of the major unmet needs of older people not only because it offers an important dimension of physical revitalization, such as improved breathing, stimulation of the cardiovascular system, toning up of the neuromuscular systems, but also because the accompanying dimension of the liberated emotional and sensual response is derived from improvisation and creative joy. One of the very major problems of the older individual is the inability to experience spontaneity and joy, to express their individuality physically, and to restore the all-important sensation of pulsating life. Dance therapy is uniquely appropriate for this healing.

It is necessary that some special training in gerontology be undertaken by dance therapists working with older people, primarily to overcome the continuation of stereotyped self-views and self-inhibiting attitudes. There is a prevailing tendency for younger people to become oversupportive in therapeutic roles with the aged. Thus, they convey an impression of condescension or lack of confidence in the ability of older people to understand their own physical limitations.

What is needed is dance therapy at three levels: (1) encouragement of body movement in any health form, through the stimulation by rhythm and music; (2) provision of a "safe" creative environment where no standards are set for performance in the conventional sense; (3) encouragement of the physical expression of emotion and fantasy and open contact with the fountains of feeling and imagination that are an inherent part of life at any age. This overcomes such inhibitions as may exist in forms of earlier repressions due to inner conflicts of religious or social taboos, plus those of the aging process itself.

A variety of techniques exist that are appropriate for the realistic limitations of aging people at the physical level, while at the psychic level, the fundamental techniques for personality assertion, emotion integration, and catharsis are as applicable to older people as to any other age group and certainly equally needed. Dance therapy for the aging offers an important field for the dance therapist and for gerontological research by professionals and by the governmental agencies associated with aging.

The dance therapist, apart from the necessity of adapting the physical techniques, must also be sensitive in two special areas: (1) in curbing the natural tendency of younger people to be oversupportive to the elderly, which is often interpreted by patients as condescension, (2) in differentiating properly between the real and the imagined problems in physical functioning.

Dance therapy, with these considerations in mind, particularly the psychomotor restructuring part of the program, is appropriate to the needs for physical activity; moreover, since such restructuring has the dance aspect, that is, movement to music and rhythms, such stimulation is conducive to responsive movement.

With improvements in balance and coordination, more courage, confidence, and enterprise appear, and a bridge is built toward socialization. Physical contact is therefore established, in terms of such nonthreatening experiences as holding hands, putting hands on shoulders, entwining arms or waists with arms, even hugging—all are part of the simple group dance movements.

The emphasis in the dance sessions is first and foremost on the motivation and joy in movement per se. According to the level of functioning of the particular group, the session might begin with forming a circle. This circle may be formed by having patients stand or sit on a chair (or wheelchair). In the latter case, the distance between the chairs will vary according to the wishes of each individual. As the session progresses, the therapist may ask the group to join hands, the first move toward making contact with one another. All along, one must make allowances for some patients who may sit on the side, unwilling, some who wander around saying hello to the group for attention, and some who leave the room. With appropriate music (and this *could be* a melody from earlier years) that is not too overwhelming, but is soothing in the background, swaying or swinging with the arms can be done, the head can be moved forward and backward and in all directions. Arms can be lifted and the body bent forward or twisted. At the forming of a circle, small steps to the sides can be made, as in social dances, and soon the whole circle can move sideways, as in a folk dance.

Beginning at such a simple movement level, it is surprising how soon one can make the sessions more interesting and also get the members' attention for the physical therapeutic processes by starting with relaxation, a significant prospect in itself, which is most needed, since it is also the beginning of all co-ordinated movement. The change from *relaxation* to *function* to *relaxation* as a conscious experience opens the door to movement on any level, for everyone.

As the sessions continue, elevation and bends strengthen the legs and feet, stretches and rotation of thorax improves digestion, balance and placement of body weight improve facility for walking. Different parts of the body are brought into play, according to the physical resources of the patient. Although impaired or disabled parts cannot be restored, the less impaired parts can be stimulated to encourage their use and function. With simple folk dancing or the dance steps chosen from appropriately mellow social dance, experiences of pleasure and gratification will renew responsiveness and interaction.

In order to make the prticipation attractive to each member of the group, the therapist will constantly keep it adjusted to their physical and psychological tolerance. This requires attention to sense the subtle signs of impatience, boredom, or, particularly, pains in some older people who may not accept their limitations but "keep going."

Overall, the dance therapy program for the elderly within their limitations and the attritions of senescence, provides a renewal of the sense of life through restimulation of the entire neuromuscular system, with its direct feedback to emotional release and the attendant constructive impact upon feelings of hopelessness and resignation. It functions as a positive force in *maintaining* the alertness, mobility, confidence, and emotional integration needed for adaptation to the impact of the later years. If better breathing, greater range of motion, confidence in balance, coordination, and greater willingness to mobilize courage and endurance is stimulated, the older person is better equipped to retain the necessary sense of individuality and competence that can prolong independent living.

CHAPTER 7

SPECIALIZED ASPECTS OF TREATMENT (I)

GENERAL CONSIDERATIONS

THE PROCEDURES FOR diagnosis, restructuring, integration, and group therapy, as reviewed in preceding chapters, constitute the fundamental approach to treatment in dance therapy. Naturally, since each patient is a unique personality, with physical behaviors that relate to the respective uniqueness of individual life experience, environmental setting, genetic and developmental formations, certain modifications in treatment procedures will occur in response to this uniqueness. Emphasis on certain aspects of treatment rather than others may shift in accordance with the needs of the patient, but overall, the treatment program will follow the general structure indicated.

Although this structure is generally applicable to patients who are functioning at fundamentally acceptable although limited levels with corresponding impact upon both psychological and worldly fulfillment, there are other conditions where pathology exists in various forms, such as in mental retardation, severe emotional illness, e.g. autism and schizophrenia, or in the diverse forms of organic impairment. Several special applications of group therapy were presented in Chapter 6. In such situations, then, we are concerned not only with the individual needs of patients but also with the limitations and potentials of respective pathological conditions, and we must make corresponding modifications of both the approach to individual treatment and the nature of the individual treatment goals.

In terms of the overall patient population, then, we are concerned with three major categories, as follows:

1. Those patients whose motor behavior indicates emotional

problems, ego defects, or neurosis but who are relatively intact physically and intellectually, where the possibility for successful therapy is indicated and where the only modifications required in the treatment or its goals are those relating to the needs of the individual's personality and his setting.

2. Those patients, child or adult, who suffer from some form of impairment, such as those who have mental retardation, neurological impairments, or sensory deficits. While dance therapy cannot, nor is it intended to, ameliorate the basic organic impairment, it is very appropriate for treating the emotional overlays produced by such conditions, which are accompanied by the frustrations and tensions of the handicap and which are intensified by difficulties in verbal communications, by loss of self-esteem, and by feelings of social inadequacy. However, the nature of the organic or developmental deficits involved do require certain modifications in treatment technique and in treatment objectives in conformance with the intrinsic limitations.

3. Those patients, child or adult, who suffer from severe emotional disturbance that can be considered more or less as psychotic or borderline psychotic conditions, and where dance therapy may be appropriate to overcome withdrawal, to develop relatedness with others, to facilitate communications and self-expression, and to provide therapeutic opportunities for the emotions, conflicts, repressions, and so on. Treatment for the emotionally disturbed obviously requires very special modifications in accordance with the specific nature of these conditions, as well as the special needs of the individual patient.

The following discussion is intended to review the various specialized aspects of treatments, both in the areas of the diversity of needs among individuals and among conditions. This chapter is focussed on the treatment of neurosis and character disorders; Chapter 8 will deal with mental retardation and psychosis.

THE APPLICATION OF DANCE THERAPY TO NEUROSIS IN ADULTS

Neurosis is fundamentally a behavioral expression of a distortion in self-concept and in the view of objective reality. A spiral is formed developmentally, where the body behavior expresses the weakened self-concept and world view, and the perpetuation of this body behavior continues to reinforce the ego defect and the perceptual distortion. In working with neurotic patients, then, the therapist is confronting a *habitual* syndrome, psychologically conceived and physically expressed and crystallized by habitual interaction.

The duration and success of therapy depends upon many factors, the most serious of which is unconscious resistance. These habitual behavioral modes have been undertaken by the patient at the unconscious level in order to protect his psychological security, even if they produce severe unhappiness or functional interference. Consequently, although there may be considerable conscious cooperation, there is always some degree of resistance to change, because a surrender of a habitual mode represents the abandonment of a preferred, unconsciously chosen method of psychological survival.

Success in dance therapy, as in all forms of therapy, is relative to the degree that this resistance can be overcome. In this form of therapy, it is best overcome by providing the patient with physical experiences that indicate how new physical behaviors can provide superior life modes for psychological survival, that is, modes that are less costly to the patient in terms of self-esteem, emotional and social comfort, and interactive functions with others.

CASE HISTORIES

In the case studies that follow, it becomes clear that the therapist is striving to create a break in the spiral of affect. The ability to display affect, that is, to act, then becomes a more significant indication of the therapeutic impact upon neurosis than the *verbalization of ideas about the act*. We view the acts of patients in the real life situation—the carry-over of gains made in the therapeutic situation to behavior in the world—

as the ultimate demonstration of the relative success or progress in therapy. In many cases we may not be able to see a significant carry-over at termination of therapy, but we will, in most cases, see *advancement* that can be used to develop further progress either in other forms of therapy or from newly supportive conditions emerging in the life situation.

Character Disorder, Passive Dependency Conflicts

Case Study A

BACKGROUND DATA: The patient was a nineteen-year-old girl, member of a small community and of the lower middle class; her parents were separated when the patient was age thirteen. Two daughters remained with the mother. The father remarried and moved to another state. The patient had little contact with father but occasionally approached him for money. Mother remained a housewife; she was attractive and dated men; she had a number of short-lived affairs that her two daughters accepted without question as a normal way of life for women. The patient's sister was younger, very intelligent, and always considered in the family context to be a "good girl," whereas the patient considered herself a "bad girl." The patient experienced considerable jealousy; in her view, the sister had effective ways of coping with the family to get what she wanted so that she was able to go on to college, while the patient either remained at home to do housework or undertook odd jobs of a menial nature. This failure to successfully compete with her sister was a source of severe inferiority feelings and a factor in the depressive behavior.

PREVIOUS TREATMENT: The patient had entered verbal therapy, with the following complaints: depression at failures in holding jobs, in pursuing an education, in improving appearance, in overcoming obesity; distress at her inability to live alone and to maintain herself and an apartment; self-hate at her sexual promiscuity because she felt unable to reject unwanted advances. She remained in verbal therapy for two years, with the therapist attempting to direct her toward her basic interests in art and dance. After the last of a series of patient failures (dropping out from dance school), patient was recommended for dance therapy, individual treatment.

DANCE THERAPY: The patient came to first session slovenly dressed but extremely eager to dance, especially her own improvisation, and she chose a Beethoven symphony as inspiration. Once she started to dance, she could not stop and continued for twenty minutes while at the same time verbalizing incessantly in an outpour of incoherent feelings during which it was impossible to distinguish significant statements. As in her verbalization, there was no organization, control, or awareness of her dance movements. Her body structure showed the same disorganization, withdrawal of the pelvis, weak spinal column, lack of muscular strength, and retraction of the head into the shoulders.

A few sessions were conducted before application of the Movement Diagnosis Tests. (See Figure 7-1.)

DIAGNOSIS: The patient had defects in body image, a compulsive need to discharge rambling feelings, poor emotional and physical control, but good reserves of creative effort and aggression that could be constructively used. The patient was basically strong physically but uncoordinated, and she was blocked in the full expression of physical effort. The blocking of movements in the torso-leg action affected her total body coordination. Control of dynamic drive was poor, but the patient was high in courage and endurance.

The overall diagnostic picture developed in the test series was that of an aggressive, disorganized, and compulsive personality, but one of effective intelligence and creativity. The two technical problems viewed as basic to treatment were the development of coordination and of control.

TREATMENT: The ensuing sessions were spent in dance improvisations, which gave the patient ample opportunity to discharge feelings of insecurity, anger, fear, and frustration in continuous, compulsive dancing accompanied by incessant verbalizations of emotional and memory material, most of which was directed towards the difficulties in the family relationships. For several months she would endlessly emote, in language and in dance, but a good part of each session was given to exercise

MOVEMENT DIAGNOSIS TESTS

Initial Tests

NAME __Case Study A__   DATE OF TESTS __Dec. 5, 1973__
ADDRESS _____   AGE __19 yrs.__
_____   REFERRAL _____
TELEPHONE _____
Prev. Exp. with Dance or Exercises: Where: __New York__
     When: __from age 10-15__
Operations or Physical Weaknesses: __none__

- -

SCORE
(Ideal) Real

__(25)__ __25__ 1. Degree of Dynamic Drive:
    1. Push chair __5__   2. Push table __5__
    3. (Stand back against wall)   Push wall __5__
    4. (Bend knees)   Push floor away __5__ Jump in air __5__

__(15)__ __6__ 2. Control of Dynamic Drive:
    1. Responses to speed __2__ 2. Simple Rhythmic patterns __3__
    3. Relaxation - - rest __1__   "Espenak Wheel"
    Obstruction Where?

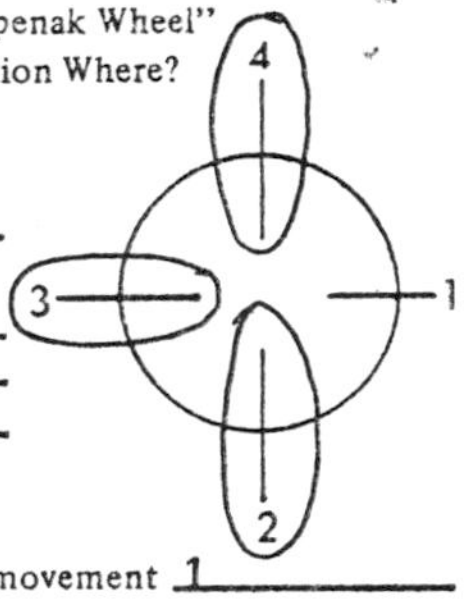

(Espenak Wheel diagram: four lobes labeled 4 (top), 1 (right), 2 (bottom), 3 (left); center labeled 5)

__(20)__ __12__ 3. Coordination:
    1. Walking and on all fours __3__
    2. Count coordinated with movement __2__
    3. Sideways walk __5__
    4. Armswings (to waltz) __2__

__(10)__ __6__ 4. Attention Span (Endurance):
    1. Hop and count __5__ 2. Driving movement __1__

__(10)__ __8__ 5. Physical Courage:
    1. Walk backward __3__ 2. Roll back on floor
    (Somersault) __5__

__(35)__ __20__ 6. Ego Image:
    1. Lift on toes __5__ 2. Stand on toes __5__ 3. Walk on toes __2__
    4. Lift arms up __2__ 5. Open arms out __2__ 6. Lift head __3__
    7. Walk on toes, head up, arms __1__

__(15)__ __15__ 7. Emotional State and Personality:
    Music stimulus __5__ Mental status __5__ Creative responses __5__

__(130)__ __92__ Total

Signed _LE_
    Liljan Espenak, DTR

For additional notes use back page

Figure 7-1.

therapy, beginning with the animal walk on all fours. Although it was difficult for her to do the progression exercises because of her sacrum problems, the patient had perseverance and showed rapid improvement.

The setting of limits was the first important step in the process of treating the lack of control and inherent disorganization. Technically, this meant that she was required to adhere to a specific theme in improvisation and would be allowed to choose images with specific content, such as *king with crown, power, arrow*, which require purposeful interpretation rather than loose themes, such as *sea* or *fire* which would encourage free dynamics.

Treatment continued in two simultaneous phases; controlled improvisation and technical correction of the body problems, in the form of special exercises and rhythms. During this period, the patient's interest in dancing was a factor in facilitating the difficult exercise work and the development of rapport with the therapist. During this period also, her energy flow increased, and the search for jobs and other outlets began. Due to her disorganization, she lost a series of jobs, and the frustration was expressed in the therapy. Her jobs usually lasted from three to six months. A victory was attained in one job that lasted eight months. The session attendance, however, was regular.

Physically, she improved in coordination and control, but other problems appeared. Her sacrum, instead of being in a relaxed state, which would allow free swinging of the pelvis, was tensely drawn inward, creating a strong arch in the back and throwing the pelvic girdle backwards in retraction. A program was developed for relaxing the lower extremities, in addition to the central program for organization and control, while still offering opportunities for the release of hostility and frustration through foot stamping and punching movements.

In this period, which was oriented emotionally toward the release of aggression with permissive acceptance by the therapist, the acting out of sexual promiscuity intensified, and the affect was carried into the sessions, with moods swinging from remorse to rebellion. This regression was interspersed with constructive efforts. The patient applied to a university and took responsibility for a job and an apartment. School work developed satis-factorily and continuity on the job increased. She saved money for a vacation in Europe. As her self-esteem grew, the indulgence in promiscuous sex decreased. The patient experienced severe loneliness, however, and expressed this in dance and verbalization.

The treatment moved toward the use of appropriate themes in improvisation, such as *stillness, out of a cave,* and *conflict.* Training in breathing was undertaken, with conscious realization of physical controls, along with the physical program in all of the specialized aspects. As body improvements occurred, there was weight loss, improved posture, and more coordinated func-tions of the legs and torso. As she began to look better, there was also growth in ego strength.

In the second year of therapy, the patient established her first significant relationship with a man and began to experience her "social feelings" and express her needs in this regard. The obsession with family difficulties had broadened to an awareness of the social interactions of life. The patient remained in indi-vidual therapy for three years; sessions were one and one-half hours weekly. She then entered group dance therapy, which gave her new opportunities to interact with her peers and to test her new resources. (See Figure 7-2 at the end of this case history.)

SUMMARY: This study exemplifies the theories and practices under discussion: the kind of problems for which this therapy is appropriate, the diagnostic evaluations, the combination of imaginative dance and demanding restructuring activity designed to resolve the diagnosed problems, the discharge of emotional conflict into expression and consciousness, and the integration of insights into conscious living. We have in this patient a strong desire to improve the quality of life and the tenacity to main-tain a rather rigorous therapy over a three-year period. It cannot be implied that all patients and all treatment programs run their course with similar consistency and progress, but this case history does indicate what can be achieved in a relatively hopeful situation by dance therapy.

The key factors in this case are that the patient was able to tolerate the anxiety generated by the experiences of change and that she had both the strength and opportunity to carry over the gains made in the therapeutic setting to the more arduous tasks of life.

The *final* movement diagnosis tests sheet (Figure 7-2) indicates the progress made since the initial evaluation shown on the initial movement diagnosis tests sheet (Figure 7-1).

Character Neurosis and Obesity

Case Study B

BACKGROUND DATA: B was recommended for treatment with a diagnosis of character neurosis. The referring psychiatrist considered her "very depressed, suspicious, hesitant," lacking in motivation and limited in intellectual and physical capabilities. He suggested that the patient needed "push, advice, drive and reassurance, and needs very much to lose weight in order to improve her physique," but he doubted that she would "be able to continue psychiatric treatment with perseverance." Psychotherapy had been terminated, therefore, with the referral for dance therapy.

The patient was thirty-eight years of age and completely dependent on a brother who paid her twenty-five dollars a week for taking care of his children. She lived in a small, cheap, rented room, to which she had moved after her parents' death. Until then, the patient had lived at home and nursed first the mother, who had died of cancer, and then the father, who died from high blood pressure and a heart attack some five years after the mother. The patient had reached the age of thirty-six years and had been "protected" in the family until then.

The effect of this trauma had left the patient paralyzed with fear of life, to the extent that she spent all her time, when not working for her brother, lying on her bed, watching TV. It was when she did not even have interest in TV that she became alarmed and sought therapy.

DANCE THERAPY TREATMENT: B first came to therapy in slacks as wide as a skirt, and a very loose sweater. She was obviously embarrassed by her shape. She weighted 210 pounds; her arches had dropped; her thighs were very heavy and appeared to be glued together; her posture drooped forward;

MOVEMENT DIAGNOSIS TESTS

Final Tests

NAME ___Case Study A___   DATE OF TESTS _Jan. 23, 1976_

ADDRESS _____   AGE _____22 yrs._____

_____   REFERRAL _____

TELEPHONE_____

Prev. Exp. with Dance or Exercises: Where:_____New York_____

When:_from age 10-15 Dance Therapy
                                                          age 19-22

Operations or Physical Weaknesses: _____none_____

- -

SCORE

(Ideal) Real

(25) 25   1. Degree of Dynamic Drive:

1. Push chair __5__   2. Push table __5__

3. (Stand back against wall)   Push wall __5__

4. (Bend knees)   Push floor away_5_ Jump in air_5_

(15) 13   2. Control of Dynamic Drive:

1. Responses to speed __4__ 2. Simple Rhythmic patterns _5_

3. Relaxation - - rest __4__   "Espenak Wheel"
                                    Obstruction Where?   4

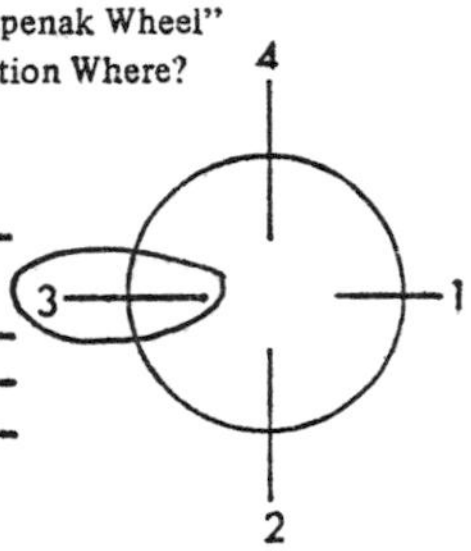

(20) 18   3. Coordination:

1. Walking and on all fours __4__

2. Count coordinated with
   movement __4__

3. Sideways walk __5__

4. Armswings (to waltz) __5__

3 — 1

2

(10) 8   4. Attention Span (Endurance):

1. Hop and count __5__ 2. Driving movement _3_

(10) 9   5. Physical Courage:

1. Walk backward __4__ 2. Roll back on floor
                        (Somersault) __5__

(35) 31   6. Ego Image:

1. Lift on toes _5_ 2. Stand on toes _5_ 3. Walk on toes _5_

4. Lift arms up _4_ 5. Open arms out _4_ 6. Lift head _4_

7. Walk on toes, head up, arms __4__

(15) 15   7. Emotional State and Personality:

Music stimulus _5_ Mental status _5_ Creative responses _5_

(130) 119 Total

Signed   ℒℰ

Liljan Espenak, DTR

For additional notes use back page

Figure 7-2.

her head hung forward, revealing an unsightly hump behind the neck. Her answers to the therapist's inquiries were limited to nodding for affirmation and shaking her head for negation.

Although passive, B was willing to undertake the movement diagnostic tests and to undergo the first series of exercises, although the work was limited by her weight and physical condition. Nevertheless, she was able to go through several activating stretches and lifts in horizontal position as well as perform simple rhythmic steps to a waltz, which she chose as her favorite dance rhythm.

In the ensuing sessions, the basic purpose of therapy was, literally, to make the patient acquainted with the fact that she was alive, that her body could move, and that she would feel this movement of her body. In this context, we made her feel how her feet touched the floor, how the thighs separate on taking a long step, how to feel her feet push the floor in order to rise on toes. These simple, basic experiences appeared to have an extraordinary effect upon her; she asked to increase her sessions from the agreed upon three times a week to six.

After this first positive response, it was possible to explain the connection between physical manifestations and feelings, indicating the parallel between her inability to push herself into work or other forms of activity. She appeared to understand that the ability to kick one's feet and legs is an essential movement in life itself. The diagnostic tests could be attempted. (See Figure 7-3.)

In the first three months, B lost 15 pounds, a very minor weight loss, but it was accomplished without dieting or medication. At this time, in order to get her to feel the sensation of kicking, we first had her kick her shoe off and feel the force of the leg thrust; we then had her walk across the floor with this kicking motion. Practice in this increased her activity from the sacrum down, and her whole walk developed the feeling of action and strength. Repeated experience in this stimulated her cooperation; the felt activity and drive in her legs gave her the drive to start dieting, and she began slowly to lose more weight. She also began to bring little "essays" to her sessions that she had written on moral, social, and emotional issues. The therapist interpreted

MOVEMENT DIAGNOSIS TESTS

Initial Tests

NAME _____Case Study B_____ DATE OF TESTS _Dec. 3. 1973_

ADDRESS _____ AGE ____36____

_____ REFERRAL _____

TELEPHONE_____

Prev. Exp. with Dance or Exercises: Where: _none_____

When:_____

Operations or Physical Weaknesses: weak gallbladder - gross obesity _____

- -

SCORE

(Ideal) Real

(25)   3 1. Degree of Dynamic Drive:

1. Push chair __1__   2. Push table __1__

3. (Stand back against wall) Push wall __1__

4. (Bend knees) Push floor away _0_ Jump in air _0_

(15)   7 2. Control of Dynamic Drive:

1. Responses to speed _1_   2. Simple Rhythmic patterns _1_

3. Relaxation - - rest _5_   "Espenak Wheel" Obstruction Where?

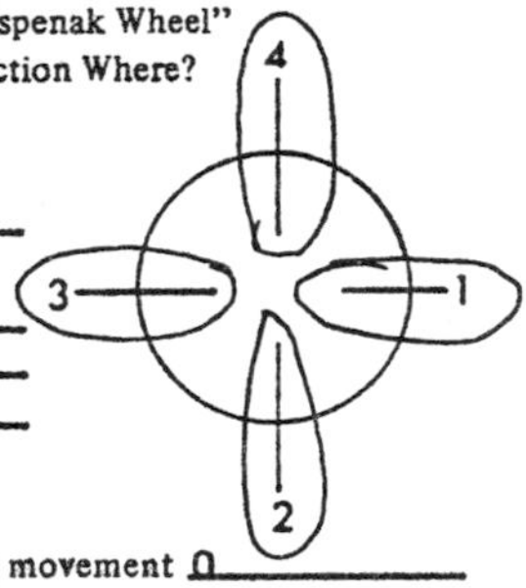

(20)   6 3. Coordination:

1. Walking and on all fours _0_

2. Count coordinated with movement _2_

3. Sideways walk _2_

4. Armswings (to waltz) _2_

(10)   0 4. Attention Span (Endurance):

1. Hop and count _0_ 2. Driving movement _0_

(10)   1 5. Physical Courage:

1. Walk backward _1_   2. Roll back on floor (Somersault) _0_

(35)   6 6. Ego Image:

1. Lift on toes _2_ 2. Stand on toes _0_ 3. Walk on toes _1_

4. Lift arms up _1_ 5. Open arms out _1_ 6. Lift head _1_

7. Walk on toes, head up, arms _0_

(15)   5 7. Emotional State and Personality:

Music stimulus _1_ Mental status _4_ Creative responses _0_

(130) 28 Total

Signed _LE_

Liljan Espenak, DTR

For additional notes use back page

Figure 7-3.

this action as a sign that the timing was appropriate to explore the dynamics of emotion relating to her arms and respiratory areas. The therapy had hitherto been restricted to the dynamics of the ordinary application of energy, developing from the sacrum through the legs, as usually employed in daily living. Now B was encouraged to lift her arms over her head, exposing the sides of her upper body and exposing her chest, which had been protected by her usual arm hug to the sides.

The performance of these movements created great anxiety in the patient. In addition to the physical body exposure, the growing mobility of the arms may also arouse a feeling or a sense of the obligations to use those arms, to *do* things. While the patient was making these great strides physically, she also began to talk about her shirking of responsibility and her dependence upon her brother. One cannot measure the role her anxiety played in the following situation, but we were informed suddenly that B was in the hospital with a broken arm. Her hospitalization, during the corresponding absence from therapy, showed both advance and regression. She made herself useful in the hospital reading to older patients and helping with the children; however, her healing was very slow because she developed a strong fear of using her arm, to the point where she even hesitated to use her fingers.

She reached the point where she recognized the psychological implications of this fear during resumed therapy and was able to continue the program of freeing the chest and the retracted head. Once she recognized the implications of her unconscious immobilization, she made great strides in the development of self-confidence, which was reinforced by the positive response in her life setting to her new attitudes. The work on her arms continued, with the objective of progressing from this to a careful approach to the problems indicated by her tightly closed thighs and drooping stomach.

Although the results of the reapplication of movement diagnostic tests indicated marked improvement in muscular response and skills, as well as in the release of aggression and the expression of ideas, she was not yet able to respond with feelings in improvisation. She had reached the point where she could move physically toward the world, but not move into it with her feelings. Her awareness of her limitations became verbal when she announced that "I have a feeling now of having my feet on the floor. I feel now I have to widen my emotional contacts, get more friends, build up my social life, and then take care of sex."

B remained in therapy for four years; she gave up baby sitting for her brother, advertised for child care jobs, and worked regularly. Her weight went down slowly but steadily to 160 pounds, and she was able to stay on a diet. She was dependable in attending sessions, both the individual therapy and the later group sessions, and developed active participation in the groups. She joined two clubs but had still to establish a direct relationship with an individual.

To take care of her social life, as she so aptly put it, she joined two social clubs, which gave her the opportunity to meet a variety of people, both male and female. It also gave her the chance of testing her own preparedness to reach out to others and expose her feelings of sympathy or otherwise.

Her sessions were then reduced to two per week with one group session, and much of this time was spent in giving her the confidence to step out in large steps and thus release the tension of the thighs. This new feeling together with the positive response she received socially made a great change in her body-ego feeling, and after another year of gradual change, she found a mate. She was then forty-two years of age. Soon after this her therapy terminated, but in following up the case three years later, B is still together with this man in a close relationship.

Although she is no longer seeking or actively engaged in any job, she is a housewife, a contributing member of any social group she belongs to, and has a full and more conscious life.

SUMMARY: In cases of obesity, the therapist is usually confronted with the refusal of the patient to move any more than is absolutely necessary to survive. The first stage of her treatment, as with all obese people, was to make her move, to convince her of her ability to operate effectively with her body and to recognize the feeling of energy implicit in movement. Moreover, for people who are trapped in nonsatisfying life situations for long periods of time, as B was, depression becomes a mode of response: the individual is unwilling to expose himself, he is unconsciously angry and consciously mistrustful. Energy is conserved for the maintenance of protective devices, and very little is left for communication or for sensory experience.

Therapeutic intervention becomes necessary to reteach with actual experience that a world of sensation lies beyond the well-constructed defenses of the patient. The immediate kinesthetic experience and its accompanying awareness evoked in dance therapy by B was the first breach of her protective armor. In subsequent sessions, her feeling of energy discharged in movement was extended to pride in accomplishment, which in turn improved the self-concept. B was not yet able to overcome her almost inherent mistrust in highly exposed situations such as sex and love relationships, but she made definitive advancement in trusting herself, which enabled her to function with more independence and positivism in the world.

The final movement diagnosis tests sheet (Figure 7-4) indicates the progress she made since the initial evaluation on the initial movement diagnosis tests work sheet (Figure 7-3).

Compulsive Neurosis and Depression

Case Study C

BACKGROUND DATA: Patient C, a sixty-year-old woman, was referred by her psychiatrist with whom she was still in treatment. She had physical symptoms, such as shaking right hand and left foot. The diagnosis on the basis of psychological as well as physical symptoms was compulsive neurosis and depression; there was apparently no determinable medical cause for the shaking behavior. C was married, and her husband assumed financial responsibility for the therapy.

DANCE THERAPY: On her first visiit, C was accompanied by her husband. She was unkempt, walked with a halting limp, had an air of "show me" defiance, and expressed her concern of being a burden to her husband because of her restriction of movement. She said she was inherently incapable of being happy and added, "I don't want to do anything. I want to lie down and

MOVEMENT DIAGNOSIS TESTS

Final Tests

NAME __Case Study B__   DATE OF TESTS __Jan. 5, 1977__

ADDRESS _____   AGE ____40 yrs.____

_____   REFERRAL _____

TELEPHONE_____

Prev. Exp. with Dance or Exercises: Where: __4 yrs. of dance therapy__

When: _____

Operations or Physical Weaknesses: __Weak gallbladder, broken left arm, somewhat__ __obese__

- -

SCORE

(Ideal) Real

__(25)__ __11__   1. Degree of Dynamic Drive:

         1. Push chair __3__   2. Push table __3__

         3. (Stand back against wall)   Push wall __3__

         4. (Bend knees)   Push floor away __1__ Jump in air __1__

__(15)__ __11__   2. Control of Dynamic Drive:

         1. Responses to speed __3__ 2. Simple Rhythmic patterns __3__

         3. Relaxation - - rest __5__   "Espenak Wheel"

         Obstruction Where?

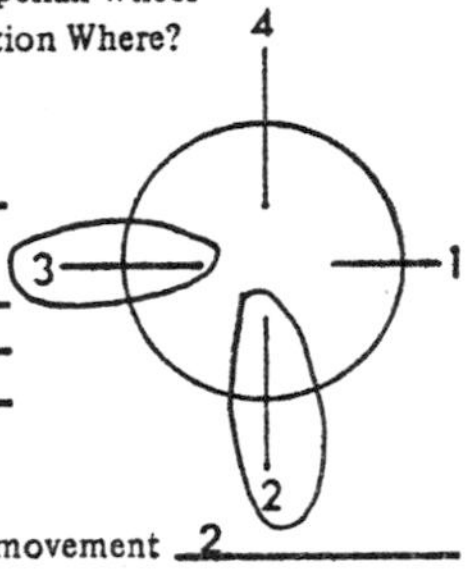

__(20)__ __13__   3. Coordination:

         1. Walking and on all fours __1__

         2. Count coordinated with
            movement __4__

         3. Sideways walk __4__

         4. Armswings (to waltz) __4__

__(10)__ __5__   4. Attention Span (Endurance):

         1. Hop and count __3__ 2. Driving movement __2__

__(10)__ __6__   5. Physical Courage:

         1. Walk backward __4__ 2. Roll back on floor
                           (Somersault) __2__

__(35)__ __22__   6. Ego Image:

         1. Lift on toes __3__ 2. Stand on toes __2__ 3. Walk on toes __3__

         4. Lift arms up __4__ 5. Open arms out __4__ 6. Lift head __3__

         7. Walk on toes, head up, arms __3__

__(15)__ __10__   7. Emotional State and Personality:

         Music stimulus __5__ Mental status __5__ Creative responses __0__

__(130)__ __78__   Total

     Signed _____

         Liljan Espenak, DTR

                     For additional notes use back page

Figure 7-4.

not get up. I am afraid of falling on my face." Indeed, an
excellent reason for the activity of dance therapy.

Her therapy began with simple stretching exercises both
to get her into a set pattern of movement and also to determine
her physical capabilities. Her muscular capabilities were generally fair or good, as were her responses to tests of kinetic
and coordination skills. Her emotional response and attention
span were very poor, however. She was obviously impatient
with the procedure and walked out after twenty minutes on the
stated assumption that the session was over.

Nevertheless, she returned. We developed a routine for
changing exercises frequently to keep her interested. Her attention span increased slowly, and she finally accomplished stretches
in all directions, arm swings to various beats, and kicks. After a
number of demonstrations undertaken by the therapist, the
patient was able to "fall on her face" on a bed, accomplished
by literally falling face forward on a soft mattress. From this
she became aware that concepts can be directly expressed in
body movement and could be dealt with directly and experi-
entially. From this comprehension we were then able to develop
the further comprehension that shaking could be a manifestation
of fear, "shaking with fear," and thus that a physical act could
reflect an emotion, conscious or unconscious.

We then worked on relaxation techniques so that the patient
could learn how to discharge energy while passive, through a
"letting go" of tensions. During the initial practice, the patient
would weep upon relaxation, but after a few sessions she became
so relaxed that she could doze for a few minutes in this release.
By the time we had built the relaxation periods up to ten
minutes, the shaking of the hand and foot began to disappear.
The patient started taking a bus to sessions instead of taxi, and
then started to walk home after sessions. During this period,
her appearance changed; her garments were clean, and she even
wore jewelry. The relaxation program became a basis for the
next advance in movement.

The limp, her most obvious symptom, was treated first. After
walking to a 2/4 march beat with the accent placed, as in the
cultural norm, on the right foot (patient's limp was in the left

Case Study C: Compulsive Neurosis and Depression

<u>MOVEMENT DIAGNOSIS TESTS</u>

Initial Test

NAME __Case Study C__   DATE OF TESTS __April 10, 1977__

ADDRESS _____   AGE ____60 yrs.____

_____   REFERRAL _____

TELEPHONE_____

Prev. Exp. with Dance or Exercises: Where:_____

When:__Social Dancing__

Operations or Physical Weaknesses: __Tremors of right hand and left foot__

- -

SCORE

(Ideal) Real

__(25)__ __14__ 1. <u>Degree of Dynamic Drive:</u>

1. Push chair __5__   2. Push table __4__

3. (Stand back against wall)   Push wall __3__

4. (Bend knees)   Push floor away __2__   Jump in air __0__

__(15)__ __8__ 2. <u>Control of Dynamic Drive:</u>

1. Responses to speed __1__   2. Simple Rhythmic patterns __5__

3. Relaxation - - rest __2__   "Espenak Wheel"

Obstruction Where?   4

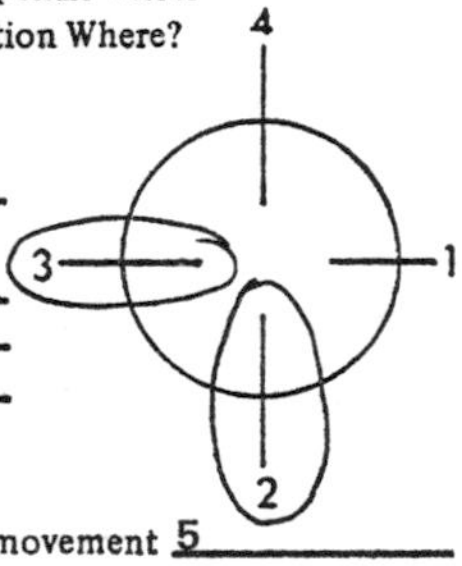

__(20)__ __14__ 3. <u>Coordination:</u>

1. Walking and on all fours __3__

2. Count coordinated with

movement __3__

3. Sideways walk __4__

4. Armswings (to waltz) __4__

__(10)__ __7__ 4. <u>Attention Span (Endurance):</u>

1. Hop and count __2__   2. Driving movement __5__

__(10)__ __1__ 5. <u>Physical Courage:</u>

1. Walk backward __1__   2. Roll back on floor

(Somersault) __0__

__(35)__ __16__ 6. <u>Ego Image:</u>

1. Lift on toes __3__ 2. Stand on toes __1__ 3. Walk on toes __3__

4. Lift arms up __3__ 5. Open arms out __2__ 6. Lift head __2__

7. Walk on toes, head up, arms __2__

__(15)__ __8__ 7. <u>Emotional State and Personality:</u>

Music stimulus __3__ Mental status __5__ Creative responses __0__

__(130)__ __68__ Total

Signed *LE*

Liljan Espenak, DTR

For additional notes use back page

Figure 7-5.

foot), she then progressed to a 3/4 beat in which the accent alternated between the right and left foot. She handled that well in the studio, but began to limp again when she left to return home. The interesting note on that limp was that she limped with the right foot, not the customary left. Disturbed from her habitual rhythms, she had simply transferred her limping device (because it was now obviously a device) from one foot to another, without being aware of it.

Her good performance in the studio steadily increased. She demonstrated her improvement in the outside setting by going to the theatre for the first time in many years, a pleasure she had rejected because "I had been unable to sit still so long." This point was reached after twenty-five sessions. The impatience was under control, and she could use relaxation techniques for control or elimination of the shake and the limp at the times these symptoms reappeared.

A second spurt of progress was made during the next twenty-five sessions. She began to walk to and from the studio and in the park. She began to read again, which was another pleasure she had given up. Her improved organization of body and mind became more and more visible in her movements and steps combinations. On one occasion she laughed, a first during her therapy, and even did improvisations on the exercises, witty versions of the movements, executed with excellent coordination.

The patient was beginning to verbalize her conflicting feelings. At one point she mentioned to the therapist her belief that "my husband is the cause of all this." Since the patient was still in psychoanalysis at that time, the therapist suggested that the patient discuss these attitudes further with her analyst. Obviously, the patient was becoming more fully aware of her hostilities toward certain dominant aspects of her husband's attitudes toward her, but she had not yet reached a grasp of the mechanisms of her own defenses and unconscious punishments in this relationship.

After a treatment duration of about six months, the dance therapy was terminated by the patient's husband. At the point of termination, the dance therapy had not been sustained long enough for the patient to surface the various conflicting elements in real depth, although some of this may have occurred in her continuing psychoanalysis. Nevertheless, the physical and social improvements she derived from her dance therapy indicated that certain constructive modifications had also occurred in her self-concept and that this ego reconstruction would be of benefit to her in holding her gains and in the possible development of stronger coping strategies in her life situation.

The final movement diagnostic tests sheet (Figure 7-6) indicates the progress made since the initial evaluation shown on the initial diagnosis sheet (Figure 7-5).

Obsessive-Compulsive Oral Dependency Complex

Case Study D

BACKGROUND DATA: Patient D was a young woman, age twenty-seven, daughter of well-to-do parents. She had a Greek background. Her father was a contractor, her mother a socialite. Her early childhood was spent in suburbia; her early life was patterned to the conventional private school and subsequent college. Family life was normal with much affection, especially for the father. She had had no previous treatment. There were no serious physical illnesses.

At the beginning of therapy, the patient was giving art lessons in private schools and maintained a relationship to a young man, also an artist. She had moved out of her parents' home in an effort to be independent and because of her relationship with the young man. Evaluation of her problems indicated the following:

1. A ravenous, uncontrolled appetite for all kinds of food, especially sweets and cakes.
2. Arguments and quarrels with her boyfriend, whom she secretly felt was not her equal, yet she was unable to react sexually to anyone new.
3. Dissatisfaction with her job, which she felt was beneath her potential.

Her mother did not approve of her life arrangements, since it did not reflect well on the family's position in the community. Her friends' daughters were already married, some with children

Case Study C:

MOVEMENT DIAGNOSIS TESTS

Final Tests

NAME __Case Study C__   DATE OF TESTS __Feb. 6, 1978__

ADDRESS _____   AGE __61 yrs.__

_____   REFERRAL _____

TELEPHONE_____

Prev. Exp. with Dance or Exercises: Where: __Social Dance__

                                   When: __10 months Dance Therapy__

Operations or Physical Weaknesses: __Tremors of hand and foot relieved.__

- -

SCORE

(Ideal) Real

__(25)__ __18__   1. Degree of Dynamic Drive:

         1. Push chair __5__   2. Push table __5__

         3. (Stand back against wall)   Push wall __4__

         4. (Bend knees)   Push floor away __4__ Jump in air __0__

__(15)__ __11__   2. Control of Dynamic Drive:

         1. Responses to speed __2__ ; 2. Simple Rhythmic patterns __5__

         3. Relaxation - - rest __4__   "Espenak Wheel"

                                     Obstruction Where? ↓ 4

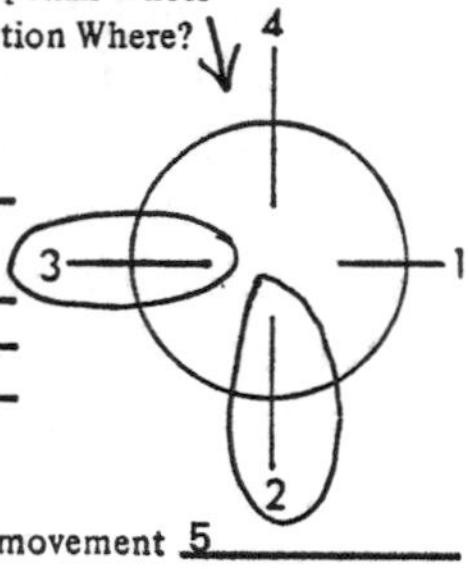

__(20)__ __16__   3. Coordination:

         1. Walking and on all fours __4__

         2. Count coordinated with

                 movement __3__

         3. Sideways walk __4__

         4. Armswings (to waltz) __5__

__(10)__ __7__   4. Attention Span (Endurance):

         1. Hop and count __2__ 2. Driving movement __5__

__(10)__ __2__   5. Physical Courage:

         1. Walk backward __2__ 2. Roll back on floor

                                 (Somersault) __0__

__(35)__ __20__   6. Ego Image:

         1. Lift on toes __3__ 2. Stand on toes __2__ 3. Walk on toes __3__

         4. Lift arms up __3__ 5. Open arms out __3__ 6. Lift head __3__

         7. Walk on toes, head up, arms __3__

__(15)__ __10__   7. Emotional State and Personality:

         Music stimulus __3__ Mental status __5__ Creative responses __2__

__(130)__ __84__   Total

Signed   _ℒℰ_

         Liljan Espenak, DTR

                        For additional notes use back page

Figure 7-6.

of their own. Those reproaches made it difficult for the patient to spend time at home, and communication had decreased to having lunch and dinner appointments with the father, who seemed to enjoy "clandestine" outings with his pretty daughter.

DANCE THERAPY: The patient had been a student of an introductory dance therapy course and so was somewhat familiar with the procedure of the sessions. She appeared in the usual professional outfit of leotards and tights, but when invited to improvise, she went completely blank and panicked.

In order to cover any embarrassment, I selected music for some Greek folk dances and improvised together with her a few simple steps. This eased the tension, and it was possible to move on to the coordination test. The patient was willing and in good health, but her coordination was blocked in several places, giving her an expression of gawkiness, somewhat as seen in adolescents in their early teens. It seemed as if her development had been arrested at this point.

Due to her timidity in expressing any emotions, we continued for a while with the physical part of our program, repeatedly working on the coordination, paying special attention to strengthening the legs for security in standing and walking. During these sessions her dissatisfaction with her poorly paid teaching job and her dependence on her father for even the slightest form of luxury were voiced constantly. She wanted legs that could "take her places," and help her "stand her ground" in life.

In venturing into the reason for her constantly low economy and quarrels with her boyfriend, she finally blurted out the most serious symptom of her problem; she would wake up at night, ravenously hungry, get dressed and go out to restaurants or drugstores, and consume enormous quantities of cakes, waffles, or pancakes. In the daytime she would carry several boxes of cookies, which she consumed secretly while at school.

Without having discovered the deeper meaning of this compulsion, we worked on organization and inner control through rhythm and dynamic exercises and succeeded in reducing the frequency of these indulgences somewhat. With the increased feeling of mastery of her daily life, her various breaks in her relationship with her boyfriend became more serious, and she

Case Study D: Obsessive - Compulsive Oral Dependency Conflict

<u>MOVEMENT DIAGNOSIS TESTS</u>

Initial Test

NAME __Case Study D__   DATE OF TESTS __May 17, 1974__

ADDRESS _____   AGE _____27 yrs._____

_____   REFERRAL _____

TELEPHONE _____

Prev. Exp. with Dance or Exercises: Where: __Sports in College__

When: _____

Operations or Physical Weaknesses: _____None_____

- -

SCORE

(Ideal) Real

__(25)__ __21__ 1. <u>Degree of Dynamic Drive:</u>

1. Push chair __5__ 2. Push table __5__

3. (Stand back against wall) Push wall __5__

4. (Bend knees) Push floor away __5__ Jump in air __1__

__(15)__ __6__ 2. <u>Control of Dynamic Drive:</u>

1. Responses to speed __1__ 2. Simple Rhythmic patterns __2__

3. Relaxation - - rest __3__   "Espenak Wheel"

Obstruction Where?

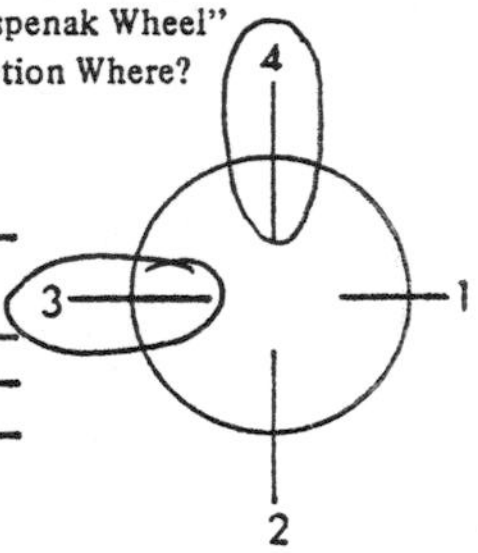

__(20)__ __13__ 3. <u>Coordination:</u>

1. Walking and on all fours __3__

2. Count coordinated with
movement __4__

3. Sideways walk __4__

4. Armswings (to waltz) __2__

__(10)__ __7__ 4. <u>Attention Span (Endurance):</u>

1. Hop and count __5__ 2. Driving movement __2__

__(10)__ __9__ 5. <u>Physical Courage:</u>

1. Walk backward __4__ 2. Roll back on floor

(Somersault) __5__

__(35)__ __25__ 6. <u>Ego Image:</u>

1. Lift on toes __5__ 2. Stand on toes __2__ 3. Walk on toes __5__

4. Lift arms up __4__ 5. Open arms out __3__ 6. Lift head __3__

7. Walk on toes, head up, arms __3__

__(15)__ __15__ 7. <u>Emotional State and Personality:</u>

Music stimulus __5__ Mental status __5__ Creative responses __5__

__(130)__ __96__ Total

Signed _LE_

Liljan Espenak, DTR

For additional notes use back page

Figure 7-7.

began thinking of making new contacts. Each time, however, she returned to the old one saying, "They (the new ones) cannot *send* me."

At one of these reports of failure she told me she was having dinner with her father, and her eyes lit up. I asked her if she could dance her feelings of looking forward to the evening. This she was able to do beautifully, revealing a very deep sensuous attachment to her father.

The next important step in the therapy came as she was asked to dance "her first memory," one of the important questions posed in Adlerian psychotherapy. In the ensuing distortions and writhings, it became very clear that this was an unconscious sexual experience. It was followed by a cathartic weeping and stammering, describing how the father came home for dinner and playfully tickled his two daughters until they were giggling and fell on their beds. During dinner time, the patient was chided because of her overstimulated appetite, and so the guilt may possibly have been born then, encompassing father, food, and sexual feelings. The eating remained her secret relating to her father.

We had hoped and half expected that with this insight our troubles would be over. But nothing of the sort happened. Emotionally, the patient fell into a deep depression, having now realized the source and size of her problem, yet she was unable to make any changes. She loved her father with all her being.

In Chapter 1, we mentioned the use of mask dances for the otherwise fearful. The possibility to identify with someone else or with the unacceptable parts of oneself, of being the boogey-man himself, or of any images one has secretly been fascinated by, in other words, to be seen but not as oneself—is a significant encouragement for one who wishes to hide his emotions. In the case of the patient, her feelings had not changed, only her understanding of them, which now made her guilt conscious. Accordingly, the masks were brought out for her to choose. There were masks of fools and devils, conceited ladies, old men, haughty kings with crown, a bird, and a donkey. She chose one of the devils, a red face with white accents and five-inch-long horns. She had danced with masks before, but at that time she could not make a choice and willy-nilly picked up a gray mousy-looking female with a stupid grin. This time she went directly to the devil and put it right on, saying half to herself, "This is my daddy." Her dance was the personification of a devil with all his wickedness, but included in it was a quality of aversion and hatred—her own reaction to what she now understood. "His eyes, his eyes," she shouted.

Now her feelings towards her father changed, and she was ready to deal with the actual day-to-day communication. At their next meeting she told him about her agony in therapy. He took it with courage and understanding. At first she would still get upset after seeing him, but gradually with cooperation, the relationship changed in quality, more towards the parent relationship to both father and mother. (Her mother stayed out of all this. The patient did not confide in her, and the father also may not have done so.)

The confusion of father-sex-food was partly cleared up. Occasional indulgence still occurred, with following remorse. But the progress attained had a greater effect on her released energies, and she arranged for studying again, taking her M.A. in art. At this time she would transgress three times per month (compared with three to four times weekly). She lived better, severed her relationship with her boyfriend without too much heartache, and was making new contacts. Still her indulgences prevailed.

Insight alone had not succeeded in changing the patient's feelings. This made it pertinent to set up a different, more direct experience of their relationship. The acting out, or directly living through movements, has always been one of the positive contributions of dance therapy. The patient's father was invited to cooperate with his daughter in this effort and based on his previous understanding, he consented.

As dance therapy theory operates with parallel and counter movements, and the emotional expression of these, the patient and her father were simply asked to begin walking from each corner of the room, to meet half way, and to pass each other. It was then apparent that these feelings were not paternal and filial. Their eyes blazed as they approached each other, and the excitement increased as they were asked to meet and then turn around and walk back to their corners. As this was repeated, some of the tension decreased. The last thing done was to meet in the center, put their arms on each others' shoulders, get eye contact, and then turn and part. I did not question the patient on her reaction. I waited for her comments. They were slow in coming, maybe weeks afterwards. "I knew," she said, "I saw it," "I am easier." It had indeed improved her self-control and feelings about herself. "He is a horrible man," she said, her aversion from before reinforced her self-assurance. Another stage in her learning of controls had been reached.

The vestige of her abnormal eating was tackled by destroying the secrecy of her indulgence. There had been two steps in the active process of organizing intake of food: (1) vomiting immediately after eating to avoid weight increase, and (2) taking refuge in devouring several heads of lettuce at a time. At her request she brought a supply to my studio to declare to the world what she was doing. (Something like the *public* confessions of some religious sects.) The rebelliousness that characterized the original drive to indulge had by now changed to a shamefacedness, which, however, was supported underneath by real strength and knowledge of self-control.

One would say now that she can "be out on her own." Meanwhile, she took her master's degree and has improved her life with qualified work in the arts, which shows promise of success and perhaps fame. Real love for a partner has yet to come.

Treatment took four and one-half years, with two sessions weekly during the first two years, then one weekly with participation in group sessions once weekly.

The final movement diagnosis tests sheet (Figure 7-8) indicates the progress made since the initial evaluation shown on the initial test sheet (Figure 7-7).

Case Study D=

MOVEMENT DIAGNOSIS TESTS

Final Tests

NAME ___Case Study D___   DATE OF TESTS ___Dec. 5, 1978___
ADDRESS _____   AGE ___32 yrs.___
_____   REFERRAL _____
TELEPHONE_____

Prev. Exp. with Dance or Exercises: Where: _Sports in College_
When: _4½ yrs. dance therapy_

Operations or Physical Weaknesses: ___none___

- -

SCORE
(Ideal) Real

__(25)__ __24__ 1. Degree of Dynamic Drive:
1. Push chair ___5___   2. Push table ___5___
3. (Stand back against wall)   Push wall ___5___
4. (Bend knees)   Push floor away ___5___ Jump in air ___4___

__(15)__ __11__ 2. Control of Dynamic Drive:
1. Responses to speed ___4___   2. Simple Rhythmic patterns ___4___
3. Relaxation - - rest ___3___   "Espenak Wheel"
Obstruction Where?   4

(NONE)

3 —— 1

2

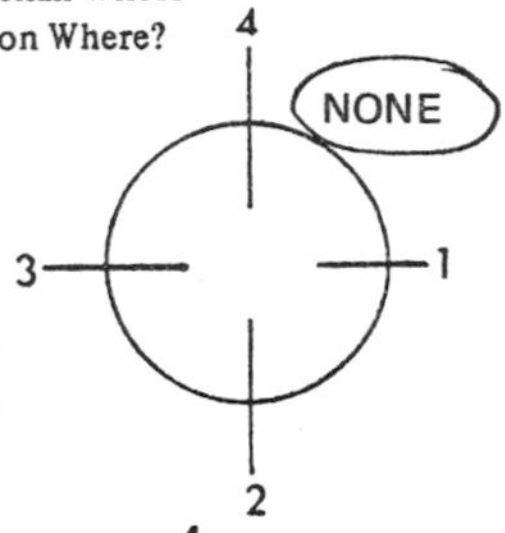

__(20)__ __18__ 3. Coordination:
1. Walking and on all fours ___5___
2. Count coordinated with
movement ___4___
3. Sideways walk ___4___
4. Armswings (to waltz) ___5___

__(10)__ __9__ 4. Attention Span (Endurance):
1. Hop and count ___5___ 2. Driving movement ___4___

__(10)__ __10__ 5. Physical Courage:
1. Walk backward ___5___   2. Roll back on floor
(Somersault) ___5___

__(35)__ __32__ 6. Ego Image:
1. Lift on toes ___5___ 2. Stand on toes ___5___ 3. Walk on toes ___5___
4. Lift arms up ___5___ 5. Open arms out ___4___ 6. Lift head ___4___
7. Walk on toes, head up, arms ___4___

__(15)__ __15__ 7. Emotional State and Personality:
Music stimulus ___5___ Mental status ___5___ Creative responses ___5___

__(130)__ __119__ Total

Signed _ℒℰ_
Liljan Espenak, DTR

For additional notes use back page

Figure 7-8.

CHAPTER 8

SPECIALIZED ASPECTS OF
TREATMENT (II)

MENTAL RETARDATION

IN THE TREATMENT OF mentally retarded children, the goals of dance therapy are appropriately modified for the respective limitations imposed by this condition. For example, the emphasis that the therapy places on independent productivity and self-fulfillment would be adapted toward more attainable ends. We would also direct our procedures toward a reduction of the disturbing emotional overlays associated with the respective handicapping conditions. We would seek to reduce certain blocks, frustrations, or inhibitions toward learning experiences so that advances in that process could be facilitated. We would seek to stimulate or improve social behavior so that the child can develop more rewarding experiences in this area and find more acceptable roles in family life.

Mental retardation itself is a complex phenomenon, with wide divergence in etiology, and it is often concurrent with other forms of handicap, such as various sensory deficits. Whether the condition constitutes a single or a multiple handicap, it is obvious that the body image and self-concept of mentally retarded children may often be inadequate or distorted, not necessarily from the retardation itself but from the emotional and social experiences occurring in the family setting, from the difficult interactions with siblings and peers, and from the confused awareness of the child of his own difference. We have here a special situation, then, where the impact of impaired function produces ego impairment, and the ego impairment reinforces the impairment in learning and in function and in socialization. Moreover, since there are limitations on the ability

131

to conceptualize and verbalize the feelings and the problems, the mentally retarded child often suffers from severe feelings of frustration without the ability or the opportunity to discharge these tensions in a setting that will accept them. All of these associated problems are reflected in body behaviors that tend to isolate the child further from the normal interactions and satisfactions of life.

Fundamentally, then, the work in dance therapy must focus upon the development of body awareness and ego strength. The movement diagnosis tests, reviewed earlier, are administered also here so that we can pinpoint the specific areas toward which therapeutic support will be most strongly directed. Technically, the treatment program proceeds along these lines:

1. Stimulating dance movements to percussion music
2. Activating movement through pushing, pulling, stretching, and swing games, played alone or in pairs
3. Encouraging individual creativity, fantasy, and emotional release through, for example animal improvisations
4. Identifying the parts of the body by touching, pointing, naming, counting, and activating, all to musical accompaniment
5. Developing coordination among limbs and other body areas to music and to rhythms
6. Providing encouragement and praise for development of a sense of self-worth by offering opportunities for physical accomplishment—an important aspect of treatment for a child who has consistently experienced inadequacy in intellectual accomplishment

This body awareness program thus combines with supportive treatment for the development of ego strength and also encompasses a learning program where certain abstractions that could not be grasped on purely conceptual terms are translated into the easily comprehended aspects of body experience, for example, shape and size differentiations; spatial and directional orientations; perceptions of difference in rhythms, tempo, and timing; perceptions of positions from different angles of vision. By using his own body as an instrument of learning, the child may learn, for example, how to form a circle with his arms or a triangle with his legs or learn to form a square with his steps, thus bypassing the difficulties of verbal and conceptual comprehension by providing the living, immediate physical experience of shapes, positions, and differentiations.

Along with these experiences in perceptual discrimination, which are conducted pleasurably as forms of play, emotional modalities are also released in sounds, shouts, cheers, laughter, and shrieks of joy or of dismay, a continuous discharge of communicative energy and feeling that often stimulates or improves verbalization. As the child participates in these experiences, he is also participating in a social relationship with the therapist and with peers, thus providing improvement in social modalities as well, strengthening both his own identity and boundaries of others.

As Director of Creative Therapies at the Mental Retardation Clinic, New York Medical College, I have worked with retarded children and with the training of dance therapists in this field for almost two decades, during which time considerable refinement of individual and group therapy techniques has taken place and to which many interdisciplinary approaches to the management of mental retardation have made considerable contribution. The total objective of the therapy, in addition to the normal goals of body restructuring and personality integration, is to provide a stronger ego base, from which the child may develop a more intact sense of self and thus proceed with stronger capacity toward the goals of his ongoing broad habilitation program.

The following case history will exemplify the current treatment program in individual dance therapy for the mentally retarded.

Moderately Retarded Child with Emotional, Behavioral, and Learning Problems

Case Study E

BACKGROUND DATA: The patient was a young girl, age fifteen, white, mongoloid, who had an I.Q. of 41, social age of 10.7, and mental age of 5 to 6 years. Diagnosis was moderate retardation—

Down's syndrome. Her parents were of good intelligence, her father a successful business man, her mother a housewife with two years of college. She had one sibling, a brother, older, of normal intelligence, good student.

The reason for selecting this case is its unusual course of development, where in a particularly difficult case, improvements and changes were also brought about through giving psychomotor dance therapy to the mother of the child as well.

E had received treatment of various kinds at the Mental Retardation Clinic, New York Medical College: medication and speech therapy, and she had taken part in two group sessions weekly, in music and dance. She had also had a series of individual sessions in psychomotor therapy by one of the students of our postgraduate course offered at the clinic. At the end of a series of twenty hours, the report said E had a few special exercises that she enjoyed over and over: *pushing* the wall, *hitting* the bull's-eye with the ball, *crawling* in competition, *fighting*. (Note the dynamics of the four verbs.)

The trainee also reported that it was impossible to have E do any motions without doing them with her. The attention-getting and controlling is obvious. She was never doing her best. With much attention given her, she *pretended* to try.

This previous report is very important because it points up how changes sometimes must be made in midstream, when the treatment approach has been unsuccessful.

Accepting our last method of approach as a comparative failure to reach E emotionally, having only somewhat improved her physical health and aggression, we decided to change the approach to a more permissive, emotionally oriented one yet remain firm with just the most necessary disciplinary limits. With these considerations, E became my patient.

TREATMENT, FIRST FIVE SESSIONS: These began a struggle that would last the rest of the year, that of developing a working relationship with E. She acted as a stubborn, uncooperative, negative, and angry child would, and she expressed these attitudes by calling names, such as "pig," trying to fight physically with me and refusing to do anything she was asked to do in the sessions.

Case Study E: Moderately retarded girl associated with emotional, behavioral and learning problems

MOVEMENT DIAGNOSIS TESTS

Initial Test

NAME __Case E__   DATE OF TESTS __Sept. 28, 1972__

ADDRESS _____   AGE __15 yrs.__

_____   REFERRAL _____

TELEPHONE _____

Prev. Exp. with Dance or Exercises: Where: __2 yrs. of dance therapy__

When: _____

Operations or Physical Weaknesses: __Mental Retardation - - Downs Syndrome__

- -

SCORE

(Ideal) Real

__(25 16__   1. Degree of Dynamic Drive:

     1. Push chair __5__   2. Push table __5__

     3. (Stand back against wall)   Push wall __5__

     4. (Bend knees)   Push floor away __1__ Jump in air __0__

__(15) 0__   2. Control of Dynamic Drive:

     1. Responses to speed __0__ 2. Simple Rhythmic patterns __0__

     3. Relaxation - - rest __0__   "Espenak Wheel"

     Obstruction Where?   4   Not available for Test.

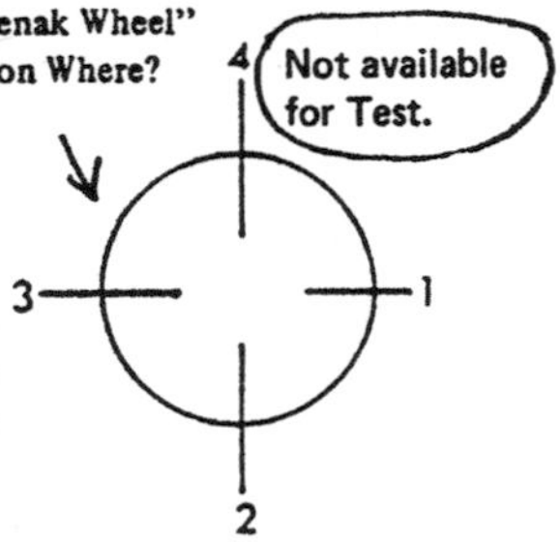

__(20) 5__   3. Coordination:

     1. Walking and on all fours __4__

     2. Count coordinated with movement __0__

     3. Sideways walk __1__

     4. Armswings (to waltz) __0__

(Espenak Wheel diagram: circle with positions 1, 2, 3, 4)

__(10) 5__   4. Attention Span (Endurance):

     1. Hop and count __5__ 2. Driving movement __0__

__(10) 1__   5. Physical Courage:

     1. Walk backward __1__ 2. Roll back on floor (Somersault) __0__

__(35) 1__   6. Ego Image:

     1. Lift on toes __1__ 2. Stand on toes __0__ 3. Walk on toes __0__

     4. Lift arms up __0__ 5. Open arms out __0__ 6. Lift head __0__

     7. Walk on toes, head up, arms __0__

__(15) 0__   7. Emotional State and Personality:

     Music stimulus __0__ Mental status __0__ Creative responses __0__

__(130) 28__   Total

Signed _ℒℰ_____

     Liljan Espenak, DTR

For additional notes use back page

Figure 8-1.

The first sessions with E indicated to me that she saw herself as an inferior person, unloved and inadequate. Her defiance was a defense against these feelings. There was no real strength backing her belligerent attitude, for her legs were very weak, with no firm contact with the floor. She held herself up with the upper part of the body. She has broad shoulders, and there was much tension from her neck down to her waist. She had trouble breathing deeply, as in suppressed emotion, and moved her arms in a mechanical way as though they were not part of the rest of her body.

During these *first five sessions*, when E broke the predetermined limits, the dance therapy session was ended, and she had to wait for her mother's return in the dressing room. Any attempt to initiate a discussion about this failed. Covering her eyes she said, "Be quiet." The therapeutic relationship seemed a long way off while we were waiting for her mother.

Always when Mrs. E. brought the child and also when picking her up, it occurred to me that she seemed very cold and unresponsive in terms of giving warmth and love to E. At the beginning of each session, E would kiss and hug her mother goodbye when she left, but Mrs. E only tolerated it, as if she did not believe E was serious.

This might be basically true; it might have been just an attention-getting device, but another mother might have reacted in a different way. All children are attention getters sometimes. She also made occasional sarcastic joking comments about leaving E "for good". In a conversation with her alone, she told me that all her friends had left her when E, a retarded mongoloid child, was born and that she, Mrs. E, had been very lonesome because of it.

A lead emerged when she half jokingly remarked that *she* ought to be having dance therapy, that she had once had dreams of being a dancer. We suggested regular dance classes for her, but her timidity would not allow her to face a class. After some consideration, it was arranged that she would have dance lessons from us. The therapeutic reason, as part of the daughter's treatment, was not emphasized but not denied. Thus, the two therapies proceeded alongside each other, the mother and daughter now having a common interest. (Reports on the mother's therapy will follow that of the daughter's.)

E especially liked being the leader, being the boss. Starting at this point the leadership was alternated, while new ways of being equal partners in movement were introduced. There were stretches and kicks. A ball was brought in, and a table was pushed from one end of the studio to the other. Floor exercises gave an occasion for much rolling and bumping. In the end, however, there was the dressing room for disciplinary ejection.

TREATMENT, SIX TO TEN SESSIONS: During the following five sessions, E and the therapist were at war. Every session was a test; how much negative defiant behavior would be tolerated? At the slightest provocation, she was out of the studio to demonstrate to her the effect she had on other people.

Technically each session began the same way; first, knee bends to strengthen the legs and then lying on the floor for abdominal breathing. Our first goal was relaxation, especially in neck and shoulders to help her concentrate on any activity. This was followed by spinal stretches to feel the lower back solidly pressed into the floor, controlling the sacrum.

Most important was E's reaction to working on her arms. In body language used in the diagnosis tests, the arms function as the means of "reaching out" and receiving: "Arms stretched out in welcome," or "Arms around mother." E had her arms glued to her sides even when imitating a flying bird. When the therapist finally faced her squarely and opened the arms saying, "I give to you and you give to me," E was so resistant that she had to be put out of the room many times.

TREATMENT, ELEVEN TO FIFTEEN SESSIONS: In the next five sessions some kind of relationship developed. E was more cooperative. Just reminding her that if she was tired and unwilling she could wait in the dressing room would sometimes get her to cooperate (behavior modification tactics).

She now allowed more physical contact. Together with the previous strengthening exercises, new movements were selected that demanded close proximity, intertwining of arms, or parallel body movements. It would sometimes become too frightening for her. Then she would begin to push or hit; however, she was able to sustain an activity longer without getting restless (ten minutes instead of two minutes).

TREATMENT, SIXTEEN TO TWENTY SESSIONS: During the next five sessions she demonstrated remarkable improvement in her general attitude. Her mother reported that E was doing better in school and was completely off all medication.

The time was favorable for helping her release her anger with aggressive striking and punching movements. A punching doll was brought in and E was allowed to hit it, throw it, and call it names. Near the end of the sessions, she put the doll to bed. She rocked him and said goodnight to him, while hugging and kissing him. At the twentieth session, I told her a story about a little girl whose only friend had left her. She made a sad face, hugged me, and said, "No, not you," and was preoccupied with touching my face gently while the story was being told.

TREATMENT, TWENTY TO THIRTY SESSIONS: During the next sessions (20 to 25), E began in a small way to demonstrate her newly discovered ability to communicate and to give and take affection. She was encouraged to move her body freely, to strengthen her muscles in the legs and abdomen, to improve her coordination and balance. A child who can move freely has also the courage to share herself freely.

In the next five sessions (25 to 30), we were able to jump and turn, to skip around in a circle, and to improvise to a record of angry music, to which she could stamp at every step to her great satisfaction. Her trips to the dressing room became no more than a threat. Her enjoyment in the dance won out every time.

Meanwhile her mother had her sessions regularly every week.

Psychomotor Therapy Report for Mrs. E

TREATMENT, ONE TO FIVE SESSIONS: The very first session with Mrs. E clearly informed us about the stress she was living under. She was tense all over and contracted in all joints. The knees were constantly bent as if bracing her weight against something, and her ankles were stiff as if trying to keep the balance. When the body is *physically* subjected to constant pressure, this is the way it would have to meet the challenge.

Case Study E:

<u>MOVEMENT DIAGNOSIS TESTS</u>

Final Tests

NAME __Case E_____   DATE OF TESTS _June 30, 1976_
ADDRESS _____   AGE ____18 years_____
_____   REFERRAL _____
TELEPHONE_____
Prev. Exp. with Dance or Exercises: Where: _4 yrs. of dance therapy_
                                       When:_____
Operations or Physical Weaknesses: _Mental retardation - Down's Syndrome_

- -

SCORE
(Ideal) Real

_(25)_ _23_ 1. <u>Degree of Dynamic Drive:</u>

    1. Push chair ____5_____ 2. Push table ____5_____
    3. (Stand back against wall)   Push wall ____5_____
    4. (Bend knees)   Push floor away__3__ Jump in air__3_____

_(15)_ _6_ 2. <u>Control of Dynamic Drive:</u>

    1. Responses to speed __2__ 2. Simple Rhythmic patterns __2_____
    3. Relaxation - - rest __2__   "Espenak Wheel"
    Obstruction Where?

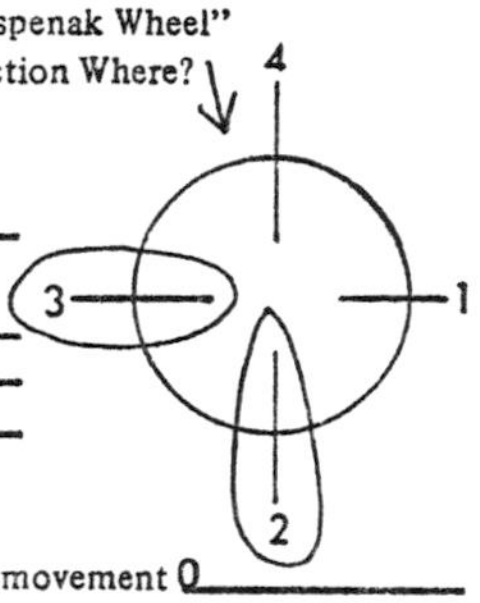

_(20)_ _10_ 3. <u>Coordination:</u>

    1. Walking and on all fours ___4_____
    2. Count coordinated with
       movement ____2____
    3. Sideways walk____2____
    4. Armswings (to waltz) ___2____

_(10)_ _5_ 4. <u>Attention Span (Endurance):</u>

    1. Hop and count ___5____ 2. Driving movement 0_____

_(10)_ _3_ 5. <u>Physical Courage:</u>

    1. Walk backward__2___ 2. Roll back on floor
       (Somersault)___1___

_(35)_ _13_ 6. <u>Ego Image:</u>

    1. Lift on toes _2_ 2. Stand on toes _2_ 3. Walk on toes _2_____
    4. Lift arms up _2_ 5. Open arms out _1_ 6. Lift head _2____
    7. Walk on toes, head up, arms ___2_____

_(15)_ _2_ 7. <u>Emotional State and Personality:</u>

    Music stimulus _2_ Mental status_0_ Creative responses _0_____

_(130)_ _62_ Total

Signed _____
    Liljan Espenak, DTR

        For additional notes use back page

Figure 8-2.

In Mrs. E's case, it was a psychological pressure, but the *body and muscles react in the same way.*

We did no diagnostic testing on Mrs. E; her sessions were intended solely as dance classes.

Our first attempts were to relax and stretch the whole body, making its inhibiting tensions apparent to her. Walking and running steps, slow and fast, high and low, with long steps and short steps, forward and backward.

TREATMENT, SIX TO THIRTEEN SESSIONS: Classes included stretches on the floor, bouncing with feet apart and with soles together. As the sessions continued, Mrs. E's emotional inhibitions came clearly to the fore. She was willing and enjoyed all movements that could be intellectually understood and described, but when it came to following any music, melody, or fantasy object, she froze up and became embarrassed. Subtle ways had to be used to approach these feelings. One of the easiest introductions to dance has always been folk dances. The music is catching, the steps can be simple or challenging, according to one's wishes and abilities. The therapist and Mrs. E did a lot of dancing and much exercise to make Mrs. E's body feel relaxed and also to trim up her figure. The physical process gave her much pleasure, and she became much freer in her expression of joy. It was evident that she, here, was receiving a most secretly desired gift.

TREATMENT, FOURTEENTH SESSION: After this, the first real response from Mrs. E was given to a Russian folk record with a waltzlike rhythm. She improvised a nice dance with light feet and used the whole space. She had good coordination and was nice to watch. It appeared she had practiced at home both technique and improvisations.

During twenty sessions the work had been on stretches and relaxation and strengthening and also "free dancing," which sounds less threatening than improvisation. Mrs. E had become aware of herself as a being, moving and breathing and dancing. Something good happened to her; she had changed. It could be noticed in her body and in her spirit.

Since she had arrived at this stage, we decided to have mother and daughter share the same therapy session, giving each of them one-half hour. First, Mrs. E would watch E having her session, then Mrs. E would have hers, and E would join her at any time. This gave E an opportunity to show off to her mother her achievements from the sessions, and it would also face her with the challenge to share with her mother or be a spectator while her mother danced.

At first the sessions were somewhat stormy, and the march to the dressing room loomed again ("time out"). Perhaps it was curiosity about what was going on in the next room, perhaps it was really the result of therapy—at any rate, E returned almost immediately to the studio and took interested part in her mother's activity, under loud criticism or praise. Both mother and daughter had a great time.

The summer vacation interrupted the sessions. E was performing on a surprisingly high level, and it was felt that we could now discontinue the individual sessions with its special attention for the time being and concentrate on demanding discipline and cooperation in the weekly group session.

For another year E was still active in this group, and the reflection of change was visible in the cooperation from E experienced in the group sessions and reported by the different departments of Creative Therapies, Music, and Dance. She ceased to step on the feet of the other children or otherwise punch them or kick them to get attention. If she stayed on the side of the group waiting for a special invitation, one request was generally enough to make her join in.

Mrs. E now has a better idea of using herself and has obtained incentive to keep working, proven because she has finally enrolled in a regular dance class. The continuation of her personal growth and the increase in her own satisfactions cannot but affect her relation with her daughter.

Due to administrative changes, therapy with E and Mrs. E had to be terminated. But, the beginnings of the new relationship between mother and daughter can develop into one of a more mutual give and take than before.

AUTISM

In discussing a severe emotional disorder such as autism, we are perforce considering therapeutic progress within the framework of limited gains. In the syndrome associated with autism, we know we are confronted, primarily, by severe withdrawal or a constellation of bizarre, highly stylized, and unique personal mannerisms and by an intensely personal and private world where comprehension and communication is more or less blocked to normal means of interpersonal access. Apart from the complex personal and perseverant eccentricities unique to the individual autistic child, there are three very major problems to consider: (1) to bridge the physical distance, the physical remoteness, as well as the emotional remoteness; (2) to moderate the aversion toward touching or being touched by another; (3) to moderate the bizarre behavior and thus open up a means of communication.

From a psychoanalytic point of view, we know that autism in children represents severe disturbance in ego formation, with consequent regression to or immobilization at a state of profoundly narcissistic fixation combined with a radical departure from reality. Moreover, this autistic personality is very defensively armored; consequently, the first task is to seek some means to develop some breakthrough in contact that will provide an opening for the development of a therapeutic relationship.

Since dance movement itself, in the preoccupation of the dancer with his own body, could be called fundamentally narcissistic and since dance, in its synthesis with music and rhythm, permits a most fluid, nonverbalized expression of inner fantasy and feeling, *dance therapy offers a particularly appropriate modality for therapeutic intervention in the case of the autistic.* If we can help the patient merge his manneristic kinetic behaviors into the dance form, we then may be able to provide a mode that is "safe" for him in the expression and communication of hitherto private ideas and emotions.

We use the symptoms themselves to draw the patient into the therapeutic relationship, often by making our own movements imitative to establish rapport with the movement language of the patient. The establishment of some form of physical rapport with an autistic personality is critical to any gains in therapy. This rapport cannot be established by dragging the patient into the therapist's reality, but only *by the sensitive entry of the therapist into the patient's world.* Therefore, by such techniques as moving with the patient, joining the movements of the patient, exploring space, distance, nearness, and direction in harmony with the movements of the patient, the presence of the therapist is tolerated, and the basis is slowly established for trust. With trust as a factor in all therapy, its development is absolutely fundamental to treatment of the autistic, since the whole question of distrust has been transformed by the patient into his nonrecognition of others.

When we talk of gains that seem so simple—the development of tolerance to presence, to nearness, to touch as these events occur in the movement therapy—we are really discussing major gains because they constitute, possibly for the first time in the life of the autistic child, a recognition by the patient that he is one of two people in a relationship, even if a word has not as yet been exchanged.

To facilitate these major events, the therapist utilizes whatever movement, activity, musical instrument, object, rhythm, or pattern that appears to be of interest to the patient so that some sharing can be initiated. Consequently, there can be little reliance on a sructured, predictable program. It is rather a matter of the ingenuity, patience, and sensitivity of the therapist to the absorptions and interests of the patient. Because of this, each case history is unique, in the sense that each patient is not only unique, as all personalities are, but he is unique in his expression of illness as well.

The following case study will illustrate a treatment approach in dance therapy to an autistic child.

Autistic Child

Case Study F

BACKGROUND DATA: F is the second son of highly educated parents; his father is an inventor and his mother is a college graduate. His brother is an important employee at a space center. F came to treatment at the age of nine, after his parents had been struggling with his schooling for the last two years.

F was classified as an autistic child. He would not make any contact with anybody; in school and at home he was silent. At home he submitted to his mother's care. In school he was obnoxious through his oblivious uncooperation, and moved from school to school in the two years from kindergarten to first and second grades.

F was untestable, and a reliable diagnosis therefore was impossible. There were no guidelines for the therapist who accepted working with him, but the mother reported that F was normal until five years of age, "When he fell out of a hammock in the garden." There were no witnesses to whether he fell on his head or even received whiplash, but after this fall F had refused to talk and functioned as an autistic child, according to his mother.

Dance Therapy Treatment: Since the Mental Retardation Center, at New York Medical College, was employing the discipline of dance therapy, it was recommended that F be sent to individual dance therapy sessions there. Accordingly, a room was selected with little furniture besides a chair and a table; and a record player was brought in with a selection of various records believed to be attractive to a little boy. No formal meeting with the boy was arranged. He was simply brought to the session after having been told that he would "be dancing."

The first time he came to the session, he promptly ran away from his mother to hide under the table. As she tried to coax him to come out, the therapist politely suggested that she leave for a while. She sat down on the chair for a moment without coaxing him, but seeing that F remained under the table where he could not be seen, she left.

F had run so fast under the table that the therapist had had no time to observe his posture or the expression of his body. She had, therefore, no indications of the personality of the patient, usually obtained through the experienced observation by the dance therapist.

In an effort to sound out the reactions to music, a record with a light beat was played ("Whistle a Happy Tune" from Walt Disney's *Snow White*). After a little while, the therapist asked F to come and join in dancing; she received no answer. The therapist played the record to its end and put another one one (a Sousa march). The volume was turned down to make the music less overwhelming, and the invitation to join was repeated. There still was no answer. The therapist danced alone and then stopped the music, just sitting down on the chair. Nothing happened during the rest of the session but soft music. The therapist did not urge F to come out, but at the end of the time, she wished him a friendly goodbye and said that she hoped to see him again.

This format of the session repeated itself more or less for the first six sessions. Occasionally F would clear his throat or tap on the table leg (not in rhythm with the music), especially when the therapist was "resting" on the chair and nothing was happening in the room. A few times the therapist thought F would join in when he tentatively peeked out from under the table, but he withdrew immediately if he saw her watch. From then on, the therapist quickly interested herself in the records and gramophone when this happened. His mother had been asked if he liked music, before therapy started. She remarked that he had a little record player of which one record was his favorite. She was asked to bring it to the session, but so far she had forgotten it. After the sixth session of the therapist's dancing to various tunes that F was likely to have heard, without having achieved any further reaction from him, the mother brought the record, and the therapist promptly played it.

The effect was stunning: F rushed out from under the table and stopped the record player. He then immediately put it on again but stopped it at the same place, perhaps after one-half minute. This stereotype behavior repeated itself over and over again, perhaps twenty times, perhaps more, in the manner of the autistic. The therapist did not try to stop it at first; she needed very much to become acquainted with F and had few clues so far. But after the twentieth time or so, she resumed her dancing to his music, and watching her move, he forgot and missed the usual place for interruption. The session ended on the usual note with "Goodbye, see you on Wednesday."

Each time after that, the stretch of music became longer and longer, F watching the therapist out of the corner of his eye. If she looked at him, he would stop the record. The session had now arrived at some sort of relationship in which he tested

her and her function. She shortened the sessions, as this tension
could not easily be sustained.

For a few times the sessions followed this pattern; after
the first run under the table, the playing of the record would
bring him out, and the strange performance would begin.

Then one day the therapist applied the rocking movement
(one of the techniques). The music was the same as before,
but the rocking movement was diverging from the pattern.
While rocking back and forth, she moved around the room as
F now sat in the chair, apparently oblivious to the continuing
record and movements, until she came up beside him, still
rocking, rocking, and rocking. For a second he moved side to
side with her ever so slightly and then sat again, turned inward.

This then became the pattern for the next two or three
sessions. The two rocked in unison, two to three times at first,
F sitting on the chair while the therapist changed the monotony
of the rocking from being sideways to being in front, actually
face to face. This was a great step forward.

F had not spoken yet and did not make eye contact, but his
eyes were following the therapist's movements, and his rocking
movements were completely in unison with hers. She could now
dare to go further and move F off his chair onto the floor, to
embrace space, facing him and by now holding his hands in
hers. They did the rocking forward and back, forward and back,
with the *forward* rocking getting gradually stronger, until it got
strong enough to pull F off his chair for a moment. Then he was
back again on the chair. Presently F was standing with his
hands in hers in the middle of the floor. The rocking continued
together without the chair for the rest of that session and perhaps
for five more sessions.

By now contact was made, and F came willingly to the
sessions; he knew what to expect and cooperated; however, he
did this with a deadpan face. The only facial expression ever
seen on his face was his furtive side look out of the corners of
his eyes. The therapist began to suspect that F was not a genuine
autistic case but an emotionally disturbed child, with strong
withdrawal symptoms. This sideways look to observe the effect
on the surroundings of his gross disinterest in anything indicated

more a resentment and passive *resistance* to authority. (Had he *resented* that the parents had not prevented his fall from the hammock? Was his attitude hostility instead of autism?)

The advantage of dance therapy or psychomotor therapy is that one can be actively working on a case through the physical approach even without a definite diagnosis because of *the physical norm available for comparison* while attempting to attain *the psychological goal through the movement action.*

A real program of dance movement exercises could now be started very, very gradually. The therapist had to be very sensitive to the boy's level of frustration tolerance, which would change with each session. The rocking now developed into swings, which when increased dynamically almost lifted him off the floor. Then the therapist saw F smile for the first time. He could now accept her touching his shoulder. With the swings in unison, her hand was on his shoulder, helping to convey directly the feeling of the lift. As he had difficulties following the musical accents given for the specific moment of the lift, she would talk in rhythm with the movement and on the impetus loudly say "up." Suddenly F said "up" loudly when she forgot it. Her efforts to develop this into "one, two, three, and 'up'" did not succeed, but he apparently enjoyed the movement, for he started the rhythm each time he came to his sessions.

After stabilizing the cooperation she was now receiving, she felt that it might be time for F to try out the group sessions. His mother had reported that he was changing his behavior in school and would follow the teacher's instruction occasionally. As there was a group dance session at the clinic every week, F was invited to come.

Time after time F would come and sit on a chair, with a blank look on his face, apparently not seeing all the activity in front of him; however, he did come and had not resisted his mother. To everybody's surprise, one day he jumped up and placed himself in the middle of the circle of dancing children. From there he watched sideways with his furtive look, just as he had done at the beginning of therapy. But, it was important; he placed himself in the center of the group. As the group was used to having a leader in the center of the circle, there was no exaggerated reaction from the children. This gave him enough time to adjust to the enormous step he had just made. Little by little he found his place in the group and would take on the leadership in suggesting movements from his experience in the individual sessions. In the circle he would soon join in with the compelling rhythm of the group movement.

F was not yet talking, but he was expressing himself with his body. He was now accessible for regular speech therapy.

Unfortunately for his dance therapy progress, F's father was offered a job in Virginia, and the family moved away. Later reports, however, told us that F had improved his behavior in school, and along with speech therapy, he was following the curriculum of his peers.

This may not have been a case of true autism, although the symptoms were such. In autism, however, the procedure runs along similar lines, mostly requiring longer duration of treatment, which makes them less suitable for presentation.

Schizophrenia

Case Study G

BACKGROUND DATA: Patient G was about eighteen when she came to therapy. She was the daughter of divorced parents. She had one sibling, a younger brother who also had psychological problems. G was a school dropout, quite heavily on drugs, defiant and negative, suicidal at times. She would not have been accepted as a patient even with the supervision available, but the application had been accompanied by the statement that she had refused all professional help for years. Apparently the dance aspect of our therapy was more palatable to her, and she agreed to come at the advice of a friend.

DANCE THERAPY TREATMENT: Thin and completely unphysical, dark eyed and black haired, stooped over with spindly legs, she appeared at the studio. One wondered how she managed to put one foot in front of the other. Her body swayed back and forth, even when standing still, and there was no contact between arms and the torso, not to mention the ground. The emotional expression of that body was nil; there has seldom been emotional starvation more clearly demonstrated. Although a vague rapport of sympathy sprang up, she had to be approached with a most delicate touch, as one does with a dog that has been whipped and shies away when you reach out with your hand to stroke it.

The first year the sessions were sporadic. More often than not she stayed away, asleep at home, or came more than one-half hour late. But, we hung on, there were no reproaches, and slowly trust developed. Most of the work until then had been the physical aspects of dancing. The diagnosis tests were administered as a part of dance technique without creating the nervous tension of "performing," and music was used for various strengthening exercises in dance form. (Results of the tests are shown in Figure 8-3.)

There was no dynamic drive, no ability to use any energy or life force for action. With no life force available, all other motor activities are impossible; this showed down the line. However, when it came to emotional state and personality, G suddenly blossomed forth. Without any physical technique, G made the most beautiful little "scenes," not through emotion but with an uncanny feeling for artistic lines and effect. This intellectual faculty was to become a great help for her motivation; moreover, it relieved her boredom.

We worked on her coordination as the first important step with a creeping, crawling animal walk on all fours, slowly rising to human walk, and bending over again to all fours. Running, leaping, and stamping came later, as the legs became stronger. Primitive rhythms and kicking a large rubber ball around the studio gave her a feeling of confidence and opened up her aggressive feelings. As always, when coordination and the feeling of power grew, the joy of the body in motion grew, followed by the satisfaction of controlling this body.

One day she went back to school! This was the first breakthrough. For two years she studied and took her degree while still in therapy on and off. We did the same coordination exercises and spatial orientation, now applied to improvisation. Emotional support in times of crisis both professionally and socially was much needed. Improvisation was attempted but was unsuccessful when relating to emotions.

Three years went by. Attendance was irregular, but she

Case Study G: Schizophrenia

MOVEMENT DIAGNOSIS TESTS

Initial Test Sheet

NAME ___Case Study G___   DATE OF TESTS __Jan. 1968__

ADDRESS _____   AGE __18__

_____   REFERRAL _____

TELEPHONE_____

Prev. Exp. with Dance or Exercises: Where: __In high school__

                        When:_____

Operations or Physical Weaknesses: __NONE__

- -

SCORE
(Ideal) Real

__(25)__ __1__   1. Degree of Dynamic Drive:

       1. Push chair ____1____   2. Push table ___0___

       3. (Stand back against wall)   Push wall ___0___

       4. (Bend knees)   Push floor away _0_   Jump in air _0_

__(15)__ __3__   2. Control of Dynamic Drive:

       1. Responses to speed _1_   2. Simple Rhythmic patterns ___1___

       3. Relaxation - - rest _1_   "Espenak Wheel"

                         Obstruction Where?

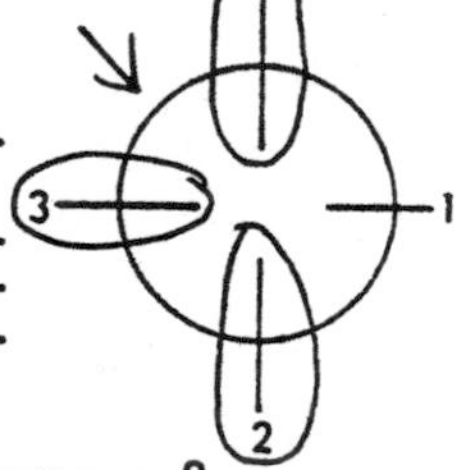

__(20)__ __2__   3. Coordination:

       1. Walking and on all fours ___1___

       2. Count coordinated with

              movement ___1___

       3. Sideways walk _0_

       4. Armswings (to waltz) ___0___

__(10)__ __1__   4. Attention Span (Endurance):

       1. Hop and count ___1___ 2. Driving movement _0_

__(10)__ __3__   5. Physical Courage:

       1. Walk backward___1___ 2. Roll back on floor

                      (Somersault)___2___

__(35)__ __10__   6. Ego Image:

       1. Lift on toes _2_ 2. Stand on toes _2_ 3. Walk on toes _0_

       4. Lift arms up _2_ 5. Open arms out _1_ 6. Lift head _2_

       7. Walk on toes, head up, arms ___1___

__(15)__ __4__   7. Emotional State and Personality:

       Music stimulus _5_ Mental status _4_ Creative responses ___4___

__(130)__ __24__   Total

    Signed _____

          Liljan Espenak, DTR

                       For additional notes use back page

Figure 8-3.

always came back. It became more and more apparent that G was unable to feel herself, and therefore, she could feel no other person either. Intellectually she realized that other people were a necessary part of her living, yet it was impossible to recognize any stirrings in herself for anybody. Life was dull, only drugs brought her a high, "Drugs make you feel yourself, drugs give you fantasy."

Movement in space and the expression of spatial directions had been a part of the sessions as our work developed. Directions from backward to forward in withdrawal and aggression and evasions sideways had been experienced, and with her intellect she enjoyed them. The question now was how to bring about the inward move, the facing of self. The circle in its repetition *allows an inward gaze while it simultaneously gives one the support of its balance.* The circular turn, mentioned in earlier chapters, through its eternally continuing rotation that does not require any new impulse, allows the consciousness to withdraw and permits that inward gaze and contemplation. So, we started the turns, very much as the dervishes do, without the ritual, of course. G turned and struggled as step followed step, cautiously determined. The movement was broken and the body divided in two, with the legs "doing their job" (aggression) and the torso (emotions) resisting the imperative circular motion. Because of this resistance against the flow, she became violently nauseous; this was also a psychosomatic method of getting out of the uncomfortable demands made upon her courage.

We modified our turns to changing sides every eight counts, which gave us seven steps to the left with one count pause on eight, and then seven steps to the right with one count pause on eight; this prevented nausea and permitted a conscious control of the turn. It also allowed for a conscious choice of tempo and degree of turn. For example, one could make the seven steps in one rotation, that is, slowly, or in two rotations, faster, or three, that is, very fast. Although there was no outright "spotting" as in the "ballet chaînées" there was a slight mental note made of the moment of spatial change. Patiently and diligently we attended to the physical, technical perfection of the controlled turns, session after session.

Dance Therapy

Case Study G:

MOVEMENT DIAGNOSIS TESTS

Final Test Sheet

NAME __Case Study G__   DATE OF TESTS __Dec. 1972__

ADDRESS _____   AGE __22__

_____   REFERRAL _____

TELEPHONE _____

Prev. Exp. with Dance or Exercises: Where: __high school__

When: __5 year dance therapy__

Operations or Physical Weaknesses: __none__

- -

SCORE

(Ideal) Real

__(25)__ __17__   1. Degree of Dynamic Drive:

     1. Push chair __5__   2. Push table __4__

     3. (Stand back against wall)   Push wall __2__

     4. (Bend knees)   Push floor away __3__   Jump in air __3__

__(15)__ __11__   2. Control of Dynamic Drive:

     1. Responses to speed __3__ 2. Simple Rhythmic patterns __4__

     3. Relaxation - - rest __4__   "Espenak Wheel"

                                  Obstruction Where?

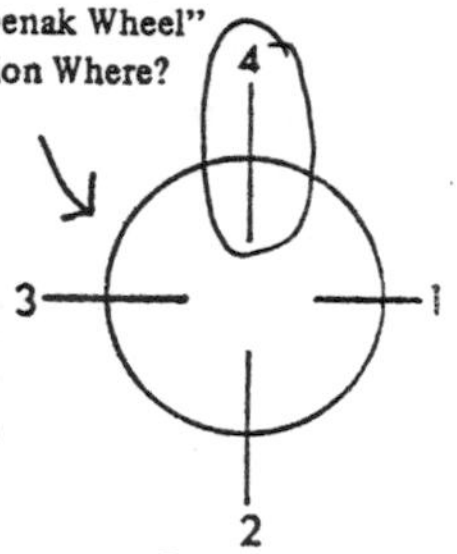

__(20)__ __17__   3. Coordination:

     1. Walking and on all fours __4__

     2. Count coordinated with

           movement __5__

     3. Sideways walk __4__

     4. Armswings (to waltz) __4__

__(10)__ __8__   4. Attention Span (Endurance):

     1. Hop and count __5__ 2. Driving movement __3__

__(10)__ __8__   5. Physical Courage:

     1. Walk backward __3__ 2. Roll back on floor

                               (Somersault) __5__

__(35)__ __27__   6. Ego Image:

     1. Lift on toes __4__ 2. Stand on toes __5__ 3. Walk on toes __4__

     4. Lift arms up __4__ 5. Open arms out __3__ 6. Lift head __3__

     7. Walk on toes, head up, arms __4__

__(15)__ __15__   7. Emotional State and Personality:

     Music stimulus __5__ Mental status __5__ Creative responses __5__

__(130)__ __103__   Total

Signed _____

Liljan Espenak, DTR

For additional notes use back page

Figure 8-4.

One day, as we were just starting, without any words, G continued the turn instead of changing sides, as if she were saying "enough of this." She turned and turned, faster and faster, almost as in anger, completely in ecstacy, until the centrifugal force became too strong and she slid to the floor, rolling a few turns as she gained support from the surface. No words were exchanged until she regained her composure and said, "That was a trip."

This was her second breakthrough. Here all our earlier knowledge of dance in history comes together with the "Medicine Man-Priest," who takes care of the tribal life, both with regard to body and soul. The primitives have always known that the body is a unit of the physical, mental, and emotional in ecstasy. It had become a perfect unit.

In each case of perfected turning, the result was a finding of self, a realization of a center, a real discovery of strength and power. Since this was nonverbal experience, little had to be discussed. The new knowledge went into the consciousness of daily living and offered not a secret place but a very private one where she could retire to be renewed and reassemble her scattered thoughts and battered emotions.

In her life she became successful in her jobs, started earning money, started also reaching out to friends, although her enthusiasm did not yet suffice to help her sustain her friendships. It was now possible to invite her to join a weekly group session. In this she was faced with the need to consider and cooperate with her peers, but she was also receiving consideration and cooperation from them. It was a give and take, and G found to her surprise that she could do both.

In observing the problems of others, she learned about her own. In the following discussions, she contributed greatly through her intellectual and aesthetic qualities, which also gave her her own particular style in improvisation. She was respected and liked by the members of the group and in time developed trust to offer her feelings of friendship. In her life she became very successful in her jobs, earning high fees and finally reaching out to friends.

Since terminating therapy, G has been climbing the ladder of success. Since her departure for the West Coast, she has been returning occasionally for reinforcement and to participate with old and new peers in the group therapy session, now an active human being in the middle of living her life.

SCHIZOPHRENIA

Undifferentiated Schizophrenia

Case Study H

BACKGROUND DATA: Patient H is a middle-aged man born in Germany of German parents during the Hitler regime. He grew up partly in orphanages and partly in foster homes, until his stepmother came to America to live and brought him along. He was then eleven years of age, went to school, and led a fairly normal life. His stepmother took good care of his physical needs but never showed any emotions or love for him. He must have been a quiet child, almost adult in his silences and depressions, who remembers sitting silently by a window with incessant rain coming down, watching the street (age seven). When the war broke out H went into the air force, which very soon proved to be more than his personality could endure, and he had his first nervous breakdown, which was diagnosed as undifferentiated schizophrenia.

From then on he had a constant history of moving from one mental hospital to another. In some cases he was placed in the violent ward. With the advent of drug therapy, H was able to receive the necessary medication to control his violent episodes, and he was released after fourteen years of hospitalization, some time before he became a patient in dance therapy. During that time he was receiving psychiatric treatment, mainly medication, and was a member of a rehabilitation clinic.

DANCE THERAPY TREATMENTS: In the first session H came into the room, pacing the floor up and down without stop. He was a compulsive walker and had no eye contact. I might as well not have been there, except for listening to his anger and despair at his long hospitalization—in bad language.

While recognizing the degree of his illness, but also partly in order to gain his attention, I, who had lived in Berlin during some of the Nazi period, began a general conversation about Germany. H was very interested in politics and well informed, and since this seemed nonthreatening, we arrived at a conversation that stopped H from moving around for two minutes during the twenty minute session. We parted, agreeing to continue our conversation next time. It took five months before H returned to the therapy session. He would disappear and appear as abruptly again without any explanation of his absences.

He might have had nine sessions in all during that first year. Every session he paced the floor, a compulsive walker as well as talker about everything and anything: his experiences in the wards, the budget problems, politics now and in history. It appeared that H had an exceptional memory for facts, dates, and places, and his brain was working incessantly, exercising his intellectual functioning. During those nine sessions, the first half was taken up with my listening to the outburst of complaint and a summary of the political happenings of the day. My contribution was mainly to listen and voice the assumption that he must feel very tense with all that on his mind. After a few sessions, I could point to the place in his neck and shoulder where the tension was located and later touch it and knead it lightly. The result of this was generally silence, but H was too agitated and tense to react for more than thirty seconds to this direct relaxation.

Unconsciously, however, it had its effect. H began to be more regular in his sessions, and it was now possible to attempt relaxation of the body on the floor. The feeling of weight and resting of the body interchanged with the "contraction-release" exercise made the feeling of tension of the body much more conscious. All his movements were performed in a jerky, violent, erratic fashion; however, he began attending sessions regularly two times per week. As time went on, the sessions seemed to have difficulty ending, and I realized that H was trying to keep me with him longer. His stream of talk was interrupted for two to three minutes at a time, as neck muscles and the crown of the head were manipulated. The relaxation treatment was continued. On the "good days" H would complete the sequences given, while on others he would just get up and leave. Still, he allowed himself to be exposed to dance therapy sessions.

It was not possible to make any diagnostic tests, but in watching H's walk there was a very notable displacement of weight from the metatarsal to the back of the heels. This creates an imbalance in the body, which is anxiety-provoking and makes one insecure. With the history of H's life, it was to be expected that he would have all kinds of fears and insecurities.

In watching his posture, the torso was leaning to the back over his heels in an expression of passivity, while the pelvic area and thighs were thust out in front of the rest of the body in an aggressive way, as if the upper body were trying to stop and hold up the aggression of the lower body. This effort had created a tight block in the area of the sacrum and hips. The head was pulled in between the lifted shoulders with a severe tension at the throat, the neck, and between the shoulder blades, just as the first approach to treatment had indicated.

With these physical problems clearly defined, it was possible to begin treatment. H needed grounding, to feel the feet grip the floor or earth, to feel the body's weight forward on the feet to prepare for the forward step, to feel the power of the back foot as it propels the body on to the front foot in progression.

H's intelligence was a great help in understanding the process, but his lack of mental control made it impossible to sustain anything for more than two minutes. Still we continued, and little by little, inconspicuously, the repetition had its effect. H started moving. The depression and lifelessness that always counteracted his violence seemed to leave him for a budding interest in being somebody, representing something. The improved feeling of the physical body paired with the relaxation of all his pent up thoughts in the head, calmed down his violence while it freed the impulse in the body for action.

Slowly, a desire arose in him to become a photographer, and with his natural talent for remembering, he wanted to be a journalist photographer. This implied a need for training and schooling of all types. We discussed these possibilities, although the goal was a long, long way off. Some purpose, though, had appeared in H's life. He came regularly to the sessions. The usual exercises were continued now with much more cooperation, and we were able to attend to posture. H had started to experience the pushing of the back foot in walking as a pleasurable feeling of control and was now interested in setting a new goal for posture.

After about fifty sessions, H was able to sit still and control his talk for almost fifteen minutes while his neck and head were being relaxed. We could now turn to the posture with some interest. Starting from the newly learned placement of the weight, we could move the torso forward with the sternum over the metatarsal. When the head also was stretched from the back of the neck upward, H exclaimed, "This feels good! I feel stronger and better." The next session he said, "I have tried out entering a room in this way, and it really makes a difference in the reaction I get."

It seemed to be the right time to move inward to emotional areas, but it was impossible to persuade H to improvise. He could do the swings and the walking as *if* he were angry or happy or fearful, doubtful, nervous as long as he was given the exact movement to make. Free improvisation was much too threatening, and it very soon was abandoned. It was decided for the time being just to counteract H's depressions and feeling of frustration. His "unworthiness" was alleviated by sharing the little he had with those who had less (or who pretended to). He gave to charitable causes and became a foster parent for a child in Africa. All these things were important for his ego. Although he definitely felt and looked better, paid off a few debts when he got his money, dressed tidily, and moved in with a girl friend, there were moments when despair and hopelessness got the better of him. Those times he just stood up and left the session after the relaxation of his head. This he no longer wished to miss.

Slowly these physical efforts bore fruit. His compulsive walking about in the sessions had stopped, and the talking disappeared. With a simple camera he walked about town and photographed the life of the city—an Irish parade, for example, with human interest pictures, beautiful old gates and doorways, and spring flowers in the parks and the streets. Mounted on a poster, the collection was impressive.

H began to excel in his chosen endeavor. Letters were written to agencies about training. Then one day he appeared at the clinic and asked for help. He had taken an overdose of medication and was taken to the hospital. (Accident or suicide attempt?) He was soon released, but the great responsibilities ahead, if he really should get well, loomed too threatening for him. He soon committed himself to the hospital again. He was still too afraid of life, of new demands made of him, of possible failure.

This time he was soon released, but his depression was overwhelming, and his eyes glassy. He moved like a zombie, and his posture had completely lost its coordination and taken on a devil-may-care expression.

During relaxation his eyes focussed a little better, and he was silent, but he suddenly rose and left. The whole long program of therapy now seemed like "crap" to him.

He attended another twelve sessions, six weeks, of obligatory appearance for therapy, relaxation, and mainly walking exercises on different levels and at different speeds. Control of dynamic force was attempted, which at first caught H's interest, since this was new. This was continued for some time in different forms to make it less boring. It was a challenge H could meet, and he improved noticeably in skill, while we unnoticeably trained his ability to control his dynamics.

The result was a sudden leap forward. Full of energy now and feeling of power through control, he went to his appointment for his training and made a favorable impression. Decisions would follow later, but he was full of enthusiasm, which carried over into the next three months. He was regular and sustained his efforts. He was interested in organizing his movements as well as his economic and social life.

Several new techniques were added, as, for instance, running with a leap and small jumps in place. The feeling of leaving the floor would have been an impossibility at the beginning. His personal hygiene and sense of clothing has improved, and he is maintaining the relationship with the girl he has lived with for the last year or so. He is much more coordinated and structured when he talks, much of which has diminished considerably, although not yet normalized. Approximately 150 sessions have taken place during which this change came about. There will continue to be good phases and bad ones, but he is now, in spite of regressions, striving for improvement and making progress for a fuller role in life.

CHAPTER 9

TRAINING FOR DANCE THERAPISTS

ALTHOUGH THE INTEREST in body therapies experienced a positive growth in the fields of psychiatry and psychology over the past thirty years, most of the work in dance therapy itself was undertaken primarily by dancers and dance educators and other specialists interested in movement both in this country and abroad. These specialists developed their personal techniques and brought their own therapeutic sensitivities and physical skills to this new and promising field. Primarily, these pioneers were individuals whose intensive professionalism was in the art of movement itself and whose personal understanding of the language of the body was expanded by undertaking serious research and study in the psychotherapeutic fields. As an outcome of the intellectual developments and emotional applications, they devoted themselves to the work with patients in those clinics and hospitals which were receptive to the possibilities of nonverbal therapies for certain appropriate emotional disorders.

In the final outcome, *their awareness, on a physical level,* paired with the thorough knowledge of *specific correspondences of the body to our specific emotions* in combination with a *physical structuring program,* today represents the important contribution made by dance therapy to the psychotherapeutic field.

One of the first major steps to professionalize specific training in dance therapy occurred in 1966 when I was invited to establish the first course for this purpose at New York Medical College in conjunction with its Mental Retardation Clinic and became the Coordinator of the Postgraduate Course in Dance Therapy, the first of its kind in the United States.

The professionalization, not only of the therapist but of the theory and role of dance therapy as a scientific discipline within the fields of psychology and psychiatry has since become an expanded endeavor in research, practice, and literature, which has been reflected in the ongoing enrichment of this curriculum. Given a positive acceptance of current proposals for introduction of *an expanded emphasis* on *psychotherapeutic education and training*, the course may constitute a model for postgraduate dance therapy training in a clinical setting.

POSTGRADUATE COURSE IN DANCE THERAPY

Objectives

1. To train dancers and dance educators in the use of dance as a tool for treatment of the mentally retarded, the emotionally disturbed, and other appropriate populations.
2. To provide the study of the theory and techniques utilized in the formulations and applications of dance therapy.
3. To provide an informed understanding of the potential and use of the dance for expression and communication.

Requirements

As previous experience with mentally retarded is not required, the objective of the course is to train dancers and dance educators in the use of dance therapy as a general treatment methodology.

Although the Mental Retardation Clinic offers a wide variety of experience with mentally retarded outpatients, the practical experience also comprises regular weekly sessions with emotionally disturbed children in the public school system, and regular weekly sessions in a state mental hospital, working with adult mental patients on the ward. Opportunities for working with the aged in a home for senior citizens is also available. All these activities provide a varied experience with different patient populations.

Applicants must have a B.A. or B.S. degree or the equivalent in dance education and must have a knowledge of several schools of dance techniques. Generally, one year of teaching experience is considered minimal. Volunteer trainees and graduate students in independent study at various colleges (Goddard, Empire State, Marymount) join in the course towards the master's degree in "The Use of Dance Therapy as a Treatment Modality."

Curriculum Content A: Clinical Training

There are weekly lectures and seminars by the staff of the clinic covering the specialized functions of the different departments from the intake by social service to the liaison with education:

1. Social service
2. Pediatrics
3. Psychiatry
4. Clinical psychology
5. Audiology
6. Physical therapy
7. Occupational therapy
8. Speech therapy
9. Music therapy
10. Art therapy

The trainees also must present their own discipline in a seminar to the staff, generally organized in the form of a panel, where certain aspects of the theory are presented by different participants, as, for example, The Physical Aspect and Training, Observation, Diagnosis Tests, Importance of Coordination, the Psychological Expressions of Body Parts, etc. The session in the public school system fosters a close contact with teachers and the school psychologist as well as with the parents, while the therapy sessions in the wards of the hospital are under supervision of the medical and rehabilitation staff of that hospital.

Each session is reported and presented for supervision and also for learning by the assembled trainees. The writing of a particular case presentation chosen from the year's experience is part of the requirements for certification at the end of the course.

A number of other papers are required, as follows:

| *Midterm*: | 15 pp. | History of Dance as Therapy |
| *Finals*: | 20 pp. | Principles and Effects of Dance Therapy |

10 pp.   Leading Groups
5 pp.   Movement Diagnosis Tests as Applied in Dance Therapy
20 pp.   Case History on Individual Patient
5 pp.   Selection of Suitable Music

During the two terms there are individual lectures given by each trainee to the assembled trainees on philosophy, based on a selected school of thought that relates in its historical development to the appropriate concepts in modern psychology, thus linking significant concepts from the age of Aristotle on to current views.

Preparation requires readings of dance theory and of the current scientific literature in the related psychological, psychiatric, and biochemical fields. (Refer to Appendix A.)

Theoretical Formulations in Dance Therapy

With the preliminary clinical orientation thus established as part of Curriculum Content A, Clinical Training and Practice, the course introduces the fundamental principles of dance therapy, organized as follows:

1. History of Dance as Therapy
    A. Dance in primitive cultures
    B. The psychological meaning of socioculture
    C. The imitation of animals and nature
    D. Function of the "coming of age" dances in primitive cultures and the parallel with contemporary culture
    E. Mask dances and their psychological utilization
    F. The expression of emotions in dance
    G. Ecstacy in dance
    H. Symbolic dancing as a diagnostic tool
    I. Religious "dancing" in contemporary life in the form of ritual
    J. The therapeutic value of the nonpictorial dance versus the picturesque dance
2. Fundamental Principles of Dance Therapy
    A. Dance as a tool of communication
    B. Catharsis through dance movement

   C. Principles of movement (body image)
   D. Body as a vehicle in space
   E. Emotional tension in muscle structure, movement diagnosis tests
   F. Structured therapy through the directed workout of specific body tensions
   G. Social and philosophical aspects

(For detail on the curriculum content of each of the preceding topics, refer to later pages in this chapter.)

   3. Kinesiology
   4. Use of Music in Dance Therapy

(For suggestions on the use of music appropriately selected for correspondence with emotional states refer to Appendix D. As a help for the trainees and also for use when beginning their function as dance therapist, this table of music compositions was created and assembled according to the special mood needed and for the expediency of the moment. It makes no pretense to be complete but only to serve as a guide until the therapist's experience can supply her with her own tried selections.)

   5. Anatomy as Related to Movement,
       Physiology as Related to Movement
   6. Field Trips
       Kennedy Center
       Creedmore Hospital
       Bronx State Hospital
       Camphill (Rudolph Steiner, anthroposophy)
       Moreno Psychodrama
   7. Film Programs (Refer to listed selections, Appendix B; distributors, Appendix C.)

A comprehensive film program shows other dance therapy approaches of the present, as well as ethnic dance films from all over the world. These films show ritual dances as well as trance dances for cathartic release but also dance as organization of communal life in its sociocultural aspect. *The emphasis on these ethnic dance films is not purely academic. It is to place dance within the psychological perspective* so that an orientation toward the profound meanings of dance for the individual and society is developed.

Curriculum Content B: Fundamental Principles of Dance Therapy

1. Dance as a Tool of Communication
    A. Psychological attitudes manifested in bodily movement habits and characteristic posture
    B. Dancing as a means of communicating on a nonverbal basis
    C. Development of body image and self-confidence
    D. The changing of self-attitudes
    E. Organization of movement
    F. Integration of movement and emotion
    G. Identification with others through cooperative activity and movements
    H. Socialization
    I. Current approaches to dance therapy
2. Catharsis Through Dance Movement
    A. The value of improvisation
    B. Releasing physical and emotional tensions
    C. The meaning and use of dynamic power
    D. Dynamics as a tool for "acting out"
    E. Imagination as a tool for "acting out"
    F. Application of emotional stimuli for improvisation
3. Principles of Movement
    A. Expansion and contraction (pleasure and displeasure)
    B. Tension and relaxation
    C. Stress-principle as energy builder
    D. Relationship to the floor (feeling push against gravity)
    E. Balance, grounding
    F. Basic principles of development of movement within the body (the wheel, the swing)
    G. Coordination in progression (the walk)
    H. The dynamics of legato and staccato (flow and vibration)

    I. Active and passive scales of locomotion

    J. Useful systems of physical education

4. The Body as a Vehicle in Space

    A. Dynamic (energy drive) as relating outwards

    B. Dynamic (energy drive) as retreating inwards

    C. Dynamics, moving into space (forward and backwards, sideways, up-down) with recognition of their psychological meaning

    D. Directional scale of the six swings (fencing principle)

    E. Symbolic meaning of the three levels (middle, high, and low)

    F. Symbolic meaning of directional patterns (circles, winding paths, squares, and triangles)

5. Emotional Tension in Muscle Structure

    A. Interrelation of emotion to muscle tension, sustained muscular contractions originating from emotion (not physical action)

    B. The importance of relaxation for achieving coordination and flow of movement: harmony

    C. Special relaxation technique—controlled falls

    D. Localization of emotional tension to specific anatomical parts

    E. Characteristic postures

    F. Diagnosis according to movement tests

6. Structured Therapy Through Directed Workout of the Special Tensions of the Body. Psychomotor Theory (Espenak System)

    A. A physical workout in parts and as a whole, answering to the particular needs of the patient

    B. Exercises for relaxing, stretching, freeing and strengthening the body

    C. Building new and positive movement patterns

    D. A workout, offering the trainees a complete personal therapeutic experience in dance therapy — control therapy

7. Social and Philosophical Aspects

    A. Systems of philosophy and psychology from Aristotle to the present

B. The most relevant schools of psychology and psychotherapy, represented by modern exponents: gestalt, reality, primal, discovery, bioenergetic analysis, Reich, Laing, and others in the constantly growing field.
C. Asiatic philosophies and their use of the physical approach
D. Family dynamics, group dynamics
E. Social conflicts, violence and addiction
F. Psychopathology, criminal and abnormal

Training Considerations

Overall, the training seeks to develop the technique and sensitivities required to help the patient achieve a needed catharsis, a deep emotional release, through acting his emotions in movement, then with the needed organization, to unify the emotional and physical behavior to the greatest degree possible for the particular individual patient within whatever limitations may exist, whether this is a pathological, neurotic, geriatric, or mentally retarded population.

Throughout the training, the inventiveness and personal sensitivity of the student is encouraged within the structure of both the academic and clinical settings, and guidance is consistently available from the professional staff in the related interdisciplinary areas.

During the fifteen years that this training program has been in operation, about 150 dance therapists have received their certificates and have entered the professional field for continued application in treatment or research.

Our work at New York Medical College, as one of the earliest sources of research and practice in the application of dance therapy, is now only one of several growing programs to augment the professionalism of the dance therapist. Considerable effort is expended today in psychology, as well as in dance therapy, to qualify and to evaluate theory, application, and results in this discipline—a broad but differentiated endeavor of considerable significance to the future expansion of dance therapy.

IMPLICATIONS FOR FUTURE DEVELOPMENT

While this book has been devoted primarily to psychomotor theory and its applications in dance therapy, many avenues remain open for research and development, both in theory and practice. To contemporary man, dance is a form of relaxation and recreation mainly for the young and is undertaken primarily in the disco form of physical isolation from the group, with occasional selective contact. Its internalized and often frenetic quality has the elements of ecstatic dance and, as such, can have its therapeutic value. It certainly has a significant function in the release of energy, aggression, and sexual strivings, along with an important focus on the pleasure of the body in action. However, in terms of authentic relatedness to others, it is depersonalized and simply accentuates the alienation of modern man in the centralized urban setting. It is thus disassociated from the mutuality of experience provided by the traditional dance forms. The communal dance requires a compact social order where there is response to the collective. It functions as a uniting and communicating agent. This collective feeling has been lost, and with it, a collective identity that is a sustaining element in human life.

The tremendous stress on man's individuality and the accompanying identity crisis experiences can be ameliorated by the therapeutic communality of group dance if it is specifically structured to meet these psychological losses and if it is appropriately adapted to the needs of different categories of people in terms of background, education, age, and interests. As our population increases, the need for reaching larger and larger groups of people in therapy becomes imperative. With his profound vision, Freud wrote the following in 1917:

> Now in conclusion, I will cast a glance at a situation which belongs to the future. We are only a handful of people and against the vast amount of neurotic misery, the quantity we can handle is almost negligible. . . . Now let us assume that, by some kind of organization, we were able to increase our numbers to an extent sufficient for teaching larger masses of people . . . the task will then arise for us to adapt our techniques to the new conditions . . . it is very probable, too, that the application of our therapy to numbers will

compel us to alloy the pure gold of analysis plentifully with the copper of direct suggestion.*

In his genius, Freud foresaw the needs for our community mental health programs, for group therapy, and for the various ancillary therapies that have been developed. In the context of dance therapy, the area of moving to music and expressing emotion on an unconscious level has an appeal and a value to many whom verbal psychotherapy and intellectualization cannot reach. The interactive nature of our inherent body-psyche-mind unity is such that developmental processes *can take place without necessarily reaching the stage of verbalized insight.*

Dance therapy also offers a direct access to body-emotion interaction, which in modern society has been blocked by the extreme emphasis on intellectualization and on purely verbal communications. With body and mind as directly interactive phenomena group dance therapy can be significant to the restoration of this natural channel. Although individual treatment, as reviewed in the previous chapters on individual case histories, is most imperative for many patients, the group approach for the "well," as well as the "ill," can provide a deeper security in dealing with oneself, and with the relationship to family, friends, work, community, and the world.

---

* **Address** delivered at the 5th Annual Psychoanalytic Congress in Budapest, 1918.

APPENDIX A

SUGGESTED READING LIST

(listed according to recommended sequence in reading)

1. Sachs, Curt: *World History of the Dance*. New York, Seven Arts, Norton & Co., Inc., 1952.
2. Lowen, Alexander: *Physical Dynamics of Character Structure*. New York and London, Grune, 1958.
3. Lowen, Alexander: *Betrayal of the Body*. New York, Macmillan, 1968.
4. Jacobsen, Edmund: *Progressive Relaxation*. Chicago, U of Chicago Pr, 1938.
5. ADTA: *Proceedings from Annual Conference*, starting 1865.
6. Chace, Marian: *Her Papers*. Chaiklin, H. (Ed.) Washington, D.C., American Dance Therapy Association, 1975.
7. Rosen, Elizabeth: *Dance in Psychotherapy*. New York, Columbia U Pr, Teachers College, 1957.
8. Espenak, Liljan: The role of dance therapy in Adlerian psychology. *The Individual Psychologist*, IV(1), November 1966.
9. Espenak, Liljan: Movement diagnosis tests and the inherent laws governing their use. *The Individual Psychologist*, VII(1), 1970.
10. Espenak, Liljan: The use of dynamics as an approach to catharsis. *ADTA Proceedings, Fourth Annual Conference*, 1969.
11. Espenak, Liljan: Body dynamics and dance as supportive technique. *ADTA Monograph*, (2), 1972.
12. Espenak, Liljan: Trance and ecstasy in dance therapy. *Proceedings from Ninth Annual Conference of American Dance Therapy Association*, 1974.
13. Espenak, Liljan: *Dance Therapy, Theory and Application*. Springfield, Ill., Charles C Thomas, 1981.
14. H'Doubler, Margaret: *Dance, A Creative Art Experience*. Madison, U of Wis Pr, 1957.
15. Schilder, Paul: The image and appearance of the human body. *Psyche Monograph No. 4*. London, Kegan, Paul, 1935.
16. Freud, Sigmund: *A General Introduction to Psycho-Analysis*. New York, Liveright, 1951.
17. Laban, Rudolph von: The educational and therapeutic value of the dance. In Sorell, Walter (Ed.): *The Dance Has Many Faces*. New York, World, 1951.

18. Kephardt, Newell: *Slow Learner in the Classroom*. Columbus, Ohio, Merrill, 1971.
19. Darwin, Charles: *The Expression of Emotions in Man and Animals*. London, John Murray, 1901.
20. Boas, Franziska: Psychological aspects in the practice and teaching of creative dance. *J Aesthetics Art Criticism, 2,* 1943.
21. Allport, G. W. and Vernon, P. E.: *Studies in Expressive Movement*. New York, Macmillan, 1933.
22. Adler, Alfred: *The Individual Psychology of Alfred Adler: A Systematic Presentation in Selections from His Writings*. Ansbacher, Heinz L., and Ansbacher, Rowena R. (Eds.) New York, Basic, 1956.
23. Adler, Alfred: *What Life Should Mean to You*. Boston, Little, 1931.
24. Dunbar, Flanders: *Motions and Bodily Changes*. New York, Wiley, 1949.
25. Kurath, Gertrude: Medicine rites and modern psychotherapy. *JAAHPER, 20*(9), 1949.
26. Gesell Institute: *Child Behavior*. New York, Har-Row, 1966.
27. Sheldon, W.: *Varieties of Temperament: A Psychology of Constitutional Differences*. Riverside, N.J., Hafner, 1970.
28. Schultz, Johannes H., and Luthe, Wolfgang: *Autogenic Training*. New York, Grune, 1959.
29. Fromm, Erich: *The Forgotten Language*. New York, HR&W, 1951.
30. Reik, Theodor: *Listening with the Third Ear*. New York, Farrar, 1949.
31. Shagass, Charles, and Malmo, Robert B.: Psychosomatic themes and localized tension during psychotherapy. *Psychosom Med, 18*:410-419, 1956.
32. Bruch, Hilde: *The Importance of Overweight*. New York, Norton, 1957.
33. Nettl, Paul: *The Story of Dance Music*. New York, Philos Lib, 1947.
34. Bernstein, Penny L.: *Theory and Methods in Dance-Movement Therapy: A Manual for Therapists, Students, and Educators*, 2nd ed. Dubuque, Kendall Hunt, 1975.
35. Bernstein, Penny L.: *Eight Theoretical Approaches in Dance Movement Therapy*. Dubuque, Kendall Hunt, 1979.

SELECTED FILMS

For film distributors see Appendix C

AMERICA AND EUROPE

Dance History, Ethnic, Folk
2 films
Part I Prehistoric and primitive dance forms
Part II Folk dance in fifteen nations
Macmillan Audio-Brandon Films

American Indian

The Long House People (23 minutes)
Rain Dance
Healing Ceremony
National Film Board
1251 Avenue of the Americas
New York, N.Y. 10020
Indian Ceremonial Dance (11 minutes)
Educational Documentary of American Indian Dances
Harold C. Ambrosh Production
Dream Dances of the Kashia Pomo (Extension Media Center)
American Indian Series
University of California
2223 Fulton Street
Berkeley, California 94720

General

Maybe Tomorrow (28 minutes)
AIM for the Handicapped
945 Danbury Road
Dayton, Ohio 45420

Movement Speaks (16 minutes)
Wayne State University
The Work Activity Center for Handicapped Adults
1940 South 2nd East
Salt Lake City, Utah 84115
Body-Ego Technique (52 minutes)
16mm, b/w
Directed by Jerri Salkin and Trudy Schoop
Darlene: A Psychological Evaluation of an 8 year old Physically Handicapped Child (37 minutes)
by Marian Chace
HC (#069-5a)
From the Inside Out (13 minutes)
b/w
Produced by Carolyn Bilderback,
RF
John: A Psychological Evaluation of an 8 Year Old Physically Handicapped Child (25 minutes)
by Marian Chace (Dr. Bice)
HC (#069-5b)
Looking For Me (75 minutes)
by Janet Adler (Norris Brock)
SS
EMC (#7782)
UEVA
Show Me (28 minutes)
16mm, b/w
UEVA and

AFRICA

Acrobatic Dance of Snake Maidens—West Africa (33 minutes)
PSU
Whirling Dervish Dance (13 minutes)
PSU
Bushclearing Dance, "GNA" folk dance—Ivory Coast (57 minutes)
PSU
N/Uu Tdiai—Trance Dance of Pushinen—Kalahari Desert, Africa
(19 minutes)

Documentary Educational Sources, 24 Dave St., Somerville, Ma.
Suite of Berber Dances (7 minutes)
Film Images, Radium Films, 1034 Lake St., Oak Park, Ill. 60301
Krieger vor Abzug zum Kampf (8 minutes)
"Dan" Ivory Coast, West Africa
PSU
Agbe Yeye (*New Life*) *Folk Dance and Songs*
Togo (a small African republic)
CF

ASIA

Dance in China (*Three Faces*) (26 minutes)
China
Chinese Information Service
129 Lexington Ave., New York, N.Y. 10016
Chinese Folk Dances—Wan-Go Weng (15 minutes)
China
Pictura Films, Distrib. Corp. 111 8th Ave., New York, N.Y.
  10011
Chinese, Korean & Japan Dance (30 minutes)
N.Y.C. Board of Ed. Audio Visual Dept., 131 Livingston St.,
Brooklyn, N.Y. 11201
Buddhist Dance of Korea (18 minutes)
UW
Sherrayattam—India (20 minutes)
Film Images—Radium Films, 17 West 60th St., New York, N.Y.
  10023
Aloha, Men's Dance (silent)
Thailand, Chieng Rai Provinz
PSU
Schwarze Lahn—Dance at New Years (16½ minutes)
(Thailand) (Tak Provinz) (Women's Dance)
PSU
Tower of Dawn, Dance of Thailand: Production Unlimited (15
minutes)
PSU
Demons & Dance of Ceylon (30 minutes)
Singhalese Folk Dances (Sri-Lanka)

Hacha, N.Y., Instructional Resources Corp. 251 East 50 St., New York, N.Y. 10022

Dance & Music of Bali (No fee) (60 minutes)

Indonesian Consulate,, 5 East 68 St., New York, N.Y. 10021

Trance & Dance in Bali

Margaret Mead—Anthropological

2 films, 20 minutes each

N.Y. University Film Library

26 Washington Square, New York, N.Y. 10012

Bayanihan Folk—Ritual customs & traditions (58 minutes)

Philippine Folk Art Center, (Manila)

Office, Philippine Consulate, 556 5th Ave., New York, N.Y. 10036

Old and New Dances of China—Taiwan (28 minutes)

Chinese Information Services, 129 Lexington Ave., New York, N.Y. 10016

Dancing of Israeli Ethnic Groups (19 minutes) Young Men's Hebrew Association, Lexington Avenue, 92 Street, New York, N.Y. 10028

APPENDIX C

FILM DISTRIBUTORS

Academic Communications Facility
   University of California at Los Angeles
   Los Angeles, CA 90024

AAHPER—American Association for Health, Physical Education
      and Recreation
   1201 16th St. NW
   Washington, D.C. 20036
ASF—Associated Films, Inc.
   666 Grand Avenue
   Ridgefield, N.J. 07657
AF—Audio Filma
   406 Clement St.
   San Francisco, CA 94118
AFB—Australian Film Board
ANIB—Australian News and Information Bureau
   636 Fifth Ave.
   New York, N.Y. 10020
BF—Bailey Films, Inc.
   6509 De Longpre Ave.
   Hollywood, CA 90028
CF—Contemporary Films, Inc.
   1211 Polk St.
   San Francisco, CA 94109
      or
   828 Custer Ave.
   Evanston, Ill. 60202
DFA—Dance Films Association
   250 West 57th St., Room 2202, N.Y.C. 10019
Dancers' Workshop
   15 Ravine Way
   Kentfield, CA 94904

DVMHF—Delaware Valley Mental Health Foundation
 Doylestown, PA
DC—Dorowite Corporation
 136 East 55 St.
 New York, N.Y. 10022
EMC—Extension Media Center
 University of California
 2223 Fulton St.
 Berkeley, CA 94720
Mrs. Magdalena Madge Gerber
 1550 Murray Circle
 Los Angeles, CA 90026
HRC—Human Resources Center
 Albertson, Long Island, N.Y. 11507 (516-747-5400)
HC—Hunter College
 Audio-Visual Center
 Hunter College
 695 Park Ave.
 New York, N.Y. 10021
IU—Indiana University
 Audio-Visual Center
 Bloomington, Ind. 47405
IFF—International Film Foundation
 Dance Films Association
 250 West 57th St., Room 2202
 New York, N.Y. 10019
Helen Lieberman, Administrator
 71 Park Ave.
 New York, N.Y. 10016
MPEMC—Mountain Plains Educational Media Council (includes
 the seven universities and colleges that follow):
  1. Colorado State College
   Instructional Materials Center
   Attn.: Booking Clerk
   Greeley, Colo. 80631
  2. University of Colorado
   Bureau of Audiovisual Instruction
   Attn.: Booking Clerk

Boulder, Colo. 80302
3. Brigham Young University
   Dept. of Educational Media
   Attn.: Booking Clerk
   Provo, Utah 84601
4. University of Utah
   Audiovisual Bureau
   Milton Bennion Hall 207
   Salt Lake City, Utah 84110
5. University of Nevada
   Audiovisual Communication Center
   Attn.: Booking Clerk
   Reno, Nevada 89507
6. Ricks College
   Audiovisual Branch
   Attn.: Booking Clerk
   Rexburg, Idaho 83440
7. University of Wyoming
   Audiovisual Services
   Attn.: Booking Clerk
   Laramie, Wyoming 82070
National Association for Music Therapy, Inc.
   P.O. Box 610
   Lawrence, Kansas 66044
PSU—Pennsylvania State University
   Audio Visual Services
   University Park, PA
PMRC—Peter M. Robeck Co.
   4 West 16 St.
   New York, N.Y. 10011
RF—Radim Films, Inc.
   220 West 42 St.
   New York, N.Y. 10036
SF—Salkin Films
   3584 Multiview Dr.
   Hollywood, CA 90028
SIP—Sandoz Ideal Pictures
   Sandox Pharmaceuticals

Route 10
Hanover, N.J. 07936
    or
Ideal Pictures
34 Macqueston Parkway So.
Mt. Vernon, New York
S-L—S-L Film Productions
    2126 No. Hartwick St.
    Los Angeles, CA 90041
SS—Shadylane School
    Department of Research
    Shadylane School
    315 Shady Ave.
    Pittsburgh, PA 15206
UEVA—Universal Education and Visual Art
    221 Park Ave.
    New York, N.Y. 10003
UCLA—University of California at Los Angeles
    Film Distributor Division
    Department of Cinema
    University of Southern California
    Los Angeles, CA 90007
UW—University of Washington
    Audio-Visual Services
    Seattle 5, Washington
WSU—Wayne State University
    Detroit, Mich. 48202

SUGGESTED SELECTIONS FOR MUSIC WITH
SPECIFIC EMOTIONAL CONTENT

ANGER (and other high degrees of dynamic feeling)

Composer	Title	Artist, Recording*	Description
Berlioz	Symphonie Fantastique (Finale)	Ormandy, Victor	agitated
Beethoven	Sonata No. 23 Op. 57	Serkin, Columbia	passionate, forceful
Brahms	Piano Concerto #2 (1st movement)	Rubinstein, LSC-2296	vigorous, robust
Chopin	Sonata for Piano	Casadesus, Columbia	dramatic, nervous rhythm
Chopin	Polonaise: Ab Major; Etude in Cb Major	Iturbi, Victor	strong, aggressive
Dukas	The Sorcerer's Apprentice	Leinsdorf, Paperback Classics	angry, strong
Ravel	Rhapsodie Espagnole	Stokowsky, Seraphim	lively, incitive
Rachmaninoff	Concerto No. 1	Richter, Monitor	passionate, strong
Rimski-Korsakov	The Russian East Overture	Leinsdorf, Paperback Classics	pompous
Wagner	Die Walküre	Toscanini, Victor	aggressive
Wagner	Lohengrin Act III	Reiner, Columbia	exciting, pompous
Wagner	Operatic Overtures (The Flying Dutchman)	Gui, Camelot	aggressive
Verdi	Aida: Grand March	Toscanini, Victor	triumphant, stimulating
Orff	Carmina Burana		strong, passionate
Moussorgsky	Pictures at an Exhibition (Gates of Kiev) Others in series also for various other moods.		pompous, majestic
Gershwin	An American in Paris		lively, dramatic (many moods)

FEAR

Composer	Title	Artist, Recording*	Description
Dukas	The Sorcerer's Apprentice	Vox Box 2, VBX -2(3-12")	anxious, threatening
Moussorgsky	Night on a Bald Mountain	Orchestra Box, Band 2	fear of nature in a storm
	Tibetan Chant, Lament for the Dead	Ethnic Folkways Library F.E. 4504, Side IV, No. 13	mysterious, dread

* Where artist and recording is not given, any recording can be used.

CALM (and other low degrees of dynamics)

Composer	Title	Artist, Recording	Description
Albinoni	Sinfonia for Orchestra (Adagio)	Stratta, RCA	spiritual, longing
Bach	Air for the G String	Toscanini, Victor	blissful, eternal, sentimental
Bach	Concerto for two violins	Stokowsky, Victor	sentimental, yearning
Bach	Jesu, Joy of Man's Desiring	Stokowsky, Victor	serene
Beethoven	Concerto No. 2 in Bb (1st movement)	Serkin, Columbia	relaxed, serene
Beethoven	Concerto No. 3 (2nd movement)	Serkin, Victor	tranquil, soothing
Beethoven	Concerto No. 4 (1st movement)	Serkin, Columbia	serious, compassionate
Beethoven	Emperor Concerto No. 5	Rubinstein, Columbia	lyrical, tranquil, light, calming
Beethoven	Moonlight Sonata (1st movement)	Serkin, Columbia	calming, repetitive
Beethoven	Piano Concerto No. 5 (Adagio)	Szell, Victor	lyrical, leisurely, serene
Beethoven	Symphony No. 6 Op. 68 (2nd movement)	Walter, Victor	gentle, steady, soothing
Brahms	Lullaby	Robert Shaw Chorale, Victor	serene, peaceful
Debussy	Claire De Lune	Stokowski, Victor	calm, tender, serene
Gershwin	Rhapsody in Blue	Levant, Columbia	broad, sentimental
Horn	Inside (Prologue) (Taj Mahal)	Horn, Epic Records	serene
Liszt	Liebetraum		intense, romantic
Rimski-Korsakov	Scheherazade Suite	Ormandy, Columbia	peaceful, calm, serene
Respighi	The Pines of Rome, The Fountains of Rome	Toscanini, RCA	calm, serene
Saint-Saëns	Carnival of the Animals (The Swan)	Primrose, Victor	meditative
Satie	Gymnopédies	Ciccolini, Angel	calm, contemplative
Schubert	Symphonie No. 8 (1st movement)	Waller, Victor	somber, restraining
Schubert	Sonata in B Flat	Schnabel, Angel	serene
Tschaikowsky	Waltz of the Flowers; Nutcracker Suite	Rodzinski, Columbia	relaxing
Valderrabano	Five Centuries of Song	Angeles, Capital	emotional, longing, yearning
Many composers	Music for Zen Meditation	Scott, Verre	calm, reflecting
Holst	The Planets		various moods
Grieg	Peer Gynt Suite		various moods of Norwegian folk characters
	Music of the Whirling Dervishes	Reinhard Anthology	calm, serene

SADNESS (longing or soothing and other low degrees of dynamics)

Composer	Title	Artist, Recording	Description
Barber	Adagio for Strings	Stokowski, SP-8673	sacred, solemn
Beethoven	Sonata No. 8 in C Minor Op. 13 (2nd movement)	Serkin, Columbia	sad, dark
Beethoven	Symphony No. 6, Opus 68	Walter, Columbia	sad, dramatic
Brahms	Piano Concerto No. 2 (2nd movement)	Rubinstein, Victor	pathetic, doleful, mournful
Bruch	Scottish Fantasy	Sargent, LSG 3205	sad, heavy, dark
Debussy	Beau Soir	Kogan, Hall of Fame	longing, dreamy
Debussy	La Fille Aux Cheveux de Lin	Sargent, LS 3205	sad, longing
Debussy	Three Nocturnes	Stokowsky, Seraphim	tender, longing
Ravel	Pavane Pour une Enfante Défunte	Kostelanetz, Columbia	low key, sad
Ravel	Le Tombeau de Couperin	Golschmann, Capital	sad, longing, resigned
Tschaikowsky	Symphony Pathétique	Karajan, Columbia	sad, depressing
Wagner	Tristan and Isolde: Liebestod	Stokowksy, Victor	depressing, dark
Franck	Fugue (No. 2) Prelude; Organ Choral No. 1		sad, melancholy
Schönberg	Pierrot Lunaire	Columbia	sad, dramatic
Stravinsky	Rite of Spring	Philharmonic, Columbia	mysterious, sad exciting, longing

HAPPY-GAY (and other high degrees of dynamics)

Composer	Title	Artist, Recording	Description
Arbeau	Orchesographie	many artists, Turnabout	happy, joyous
Bach	Six Brandenburg Concerti	Reiner, Entre	allegro, lively
Bach	Suite No. 2 in B minor	Ansermet, London	gay, happy
Barber	Sinfonia, Sacra	Hanson, Mercury	pompous, hymnal
Beethoven	Symphony No. 5 in C minor (1st movement)	Koussevitzky, Columbia	anxious expectation resolving in a stimulating and exciting conclusion
Beethoven	Symphony No. 5 in C minor (4th movement)	Walter, Victor	strong, exciting
Beethoven	Symphony No. 7 (1st movement)	Ormandy, Columbia	merry, gay, triumphant
Brahms	Symphony No. 4 in E minor (4th movement)	Walter, Columbia	optimistic, lyrical, crisp

HAPPY-GAY (and other high degrees of dynamics) (Continued)

Composer	Title	Artist, Recording	Description
Chopin	Chopin Piano Music: polonaise, waltz, mazurka	Horowitz, RCA	pompous, happy
Chopin	Polonaise in A♭ major	Iturbi, Victor	vigorous dance rhythms, proud
Debussy	Golliwogs Cake Walk	Kapell, Victor	humorous, jolly
De Falla	Ritual Fire Dance	Iturbi, Victor	surging, stimulating, exotic, driving rhythm
			exciting, warm
Dvorak	Humoresque	Kreisler, Victor	exuberant, joyous
Gershwin	An American in Paris	Bernstein, Victor	happy, gay
Grieg	Wedding Day at Troldhaugen	Remortel, Vox	triumphant, vigorous
Handel	The Messiah—Hallelujah Chorus	Beecham, Victor	garish, brilliant
Liszt	Mefisto Waltz	Kappel, Victor	bright, vivacious
Mendelssohn	A Midsummer Night's Dream (Scherzo)	Walter, Columbia	lively, gay
		Wagner, Vox	lyrical, graceful, happy
Mozart	German Dances	Schnabel, Angel	stimulating, joyous
Mozart	Quartet in G minor	Reiner, Columbia	breathless, brilliant, joyous, gay
Mozart	Symphonies: Symphony No. 35 in D major	Feidelman, Boston Pops	joyous, stimulating
Paganini	Moto Perpetuo	Colling, Decca	happy, joyous, uplifting
Sousa	Marches: Washington Post March	Muchinger, London	happy
Vivaldi	The Four Seasons		joyous, gay
Stravinsky	Early Compositions	I and II records	lively, gay
Moisetwich	Russian Folk Dances		happy rhythmical
Rodgers	The King & I (March of Siamese Children, Whistle a Happy Tune)		lyrical, graceful
Lerner	My Fair Lady (I could have danced all night)	Scherzo	bright, vivacious, lively, gay
Mendelssohn	A Midsummer Night's Dream (waltzes, Blue Danube and all others)		

MISCELLANEOUS

	Eight Electronic Pieces	Dockstader, Folkways	unemotional
	Electronic Music, Gargoyles and others	Columbia	descriptive, images
	Rail Dynamics—Recorded on Rainy Nights	Cooks	monotonous
	The Storm and The Sea	Miller, Warner Bros.	nature sounds

EXCITING, RESTLESS

Composer	Title	Artist, Recording	Description
Berlioz	Symphonie Phantastique	Columbia	exciting
De Falla	Ritual Fire Dance; Spanish Dances		ecstatic, cresendo
Debussy	Le Mer	Ormandy Philadelphia Orchestra	restless
Rimski-Korsakov	Bumble Bee	N.Y. Phil. Columbia	monotone
Stravinsky	Firebird Suite	Vox Box 2, VBX-2(3-12")	exciting phantastic
Moussorgsky	Night on a Bald Mountain	Orchestra Box, Band 2	

FOLK MUSIC

Title	Company
African Drums	Ethnic Folkways
The Azuma Kabuki	Columbia
Hukilau Hulas	GNP
Music of Bali	Westminster
Music of India	Odeon
Olatunji, Drums of Passion	Columbia
Polka Party	Golden Tone
New Folk Dances of Israel	Tikua
Russian Folk Ballet Company	Epic
The Many Voices of Miriam Makeba	KAPP

SOCIAL DANCING

Title	Artist	Company
Boogie Woogie	Freddie Slack	Wing
Bossa Nova and the New Swinging Samba	Stan Fields	Strand
Country Dances, Beethoven		
Cheganca	The Wanderley Trio	Verve
Folklore	The City Preachers	London

SOCIAL DANCING (Continued)

Title	Artist	Company
French Dances of the Renaissance and other pieces of the Renaissance and Baroque	Many composers	Nonesuch
Hi-Fi-esta	Edmunds Ross	London
Lou Reed Berlin	Lou Reed	RCA
Mantovani plays Strauss Waltzes	Mantovani	London
Medieval Renaissance & Baroque Recorder Music	Many composers	Classic
Masters of Early Keyboard Music (English Dances)	John Bull	London
Overtures and Waltzes	Moralt	Epic
Spirituals and Blues	Josh White	The Elektra Corporation

MUSIC WHEN TEACHING DANCE CLASSES

Title	Artist	Recording
Ballet Music (Vol. 1)	John Childs	Hoctor
Ballet Music (Vol. 2)	John Childs	Hoctor
Ballet Music for the Classroom	Tisen	Hoctor
Ballet Music for Barre-Centre and Six Beautiful Variations (Vol. 1)	Many artists	Statler
First Lessons in Creative Movement, Espenak	Anderson	Q.T—Records (Statler Records Corp.)
Jazz with Luigi	Fischoff	HLP
Music for Contemporary Dance	Lubin	S & R
On Stage Tap	Selva-Ringle	S & R
Paul Draper on Tap	Perkinson	H & R
The Music of Richard Rodgers	Many artists	Moodsville
African Drums—Percussion		Ethnic Folkways
Monks of Western Priory	Toni Mitchell Tim Buckley—Rock B. J. Thomas	
Hookahs and Houris	Folk Artists	Nina Records

INDEX

A

Accommodation in group dance
    therapy, 93-94
"Activity" technique, 6
Adlerian psychiatry, 38, 63
African dance (films), 173-74
Alexander technique, 37
"Analysis from below," 6
Anger and aggression, 13-16, 20, 180
Anxiety reduction, 9-10, 97-100
Appropriateness of dance therapy,
    40-41
Arm swings, 72-78
Asian dance (films), 174-75
Attachment, 95
Autism, 141-48
Avoidance, 80

B

Balance, 71-72
Bali "sitting dance," 15, 175
Ballet, classical, 19
Behavior, in movement, 43. *See also*
    Diagnostic tests
Betrayal of the Body (Lowen), 27-28
Bioenergetic Therapy, ix, 98
Biofeedback, 28
Biology of pleasure and displeasure, 61
Biped walk, 48, 65
Blockages. *See* Inhibition
Bode, 37, 63
Body
    ideal, 35
    image, 24-33, 53-54
    movement
        diagnostic tests of, 43-57, 60
        relation of sensory organs to, 33-38
    symbolic representation of, 85-86
    types and their resources, 42-43

Breathing
    cramping of, 31
    and personal rhythms, 46, 84-85
    regulation of, 21, 74, 76
Bulgarian Fire Dance, 15

C

Calm, 16-17, 21, 181
Carnival, 18
Case histories of dance therapy
    in autism, 143-48
    in character disorder with passive
        dependency conflicts, 107-113
    in character neurosis and obesity,
        112, 114-18
    in compulsive neurosis and
        depression, 118, 120-24
    in group therapy for high-risk
        patients, 97-100
    in moderate mental retardation,
        133-41
    in an obsessive-compulsive oral
        dependency complex, 123,
        129-30
    about overcoming language barriers,
        96-97
    in schizophrenia and undifferentiated
        schizophrenia, 148-59
Catharsis, 13-14, 167
Cellular reaction to pleasure, 61
Character disorder case history,
    107-113
Character neurosis case history, 112,
    114-18
Chest problems, 31, 47, 55
Classical ballet, 19
Cleveland, S., 28
Clinical diagnosis of somatic images,
    30-33. *See also* Movement
    diagnosis tests

NOV